DO it for Denim!

The
DENIM
DIET

for

ics

Th...   re

be...,3 !

Mark...ly!

Belly!

Kami

D0001949

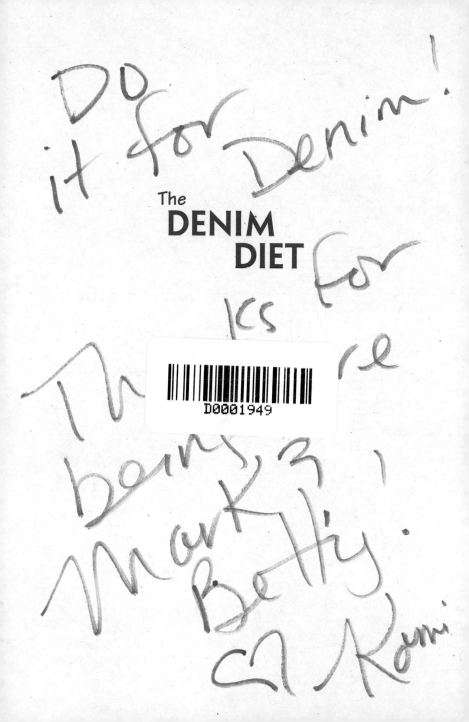

The DENIM DIET

16 SIMPLE HABITS TO GET YOU INTO YOUR DREAM PAIR OF JEANS

KAMI GRAY

New World Library
Novato, California

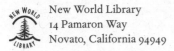 New World Library
14 Pamaron Way
Novato, California 94949

Text design by Tona Pearce Myers

Library of Congress Cataloging-in-Publication Data
Gray, Kami.
The denim diet : 16 simple habits to get you into your dream pair of jeans / Kami Gray.
   p.   cm.
Includes bibliographical references and index.
ISBN 978-1-57731-661-9 (pbk. : alk. paper)
1. Nutrition. 2. Diet. 3. Reducing diets. I. Title.
TX551.G684 2009
613.2—dc22   2008052769

First printing, March 2009
ISBN 978-1-57731-661-9

Printed in Canada on 100% postconsumer-waste recycled paper

g New World Library is a proud member of the Green Press Initiative.

10   9   8   7   6   5   4   3   2   1

TO MY PARENTS, STEVE AND KATHRYN —
THE BEST TEACHERS LEAD QUIETLY BY EXAMPLE,
WANTING NOTHING MORE THAN TO SPREAD GOODNESS

CONTENTS

INTRODUCTION

IN 1986, I WAS OBSESSED with Molly Ringwald in *Pretty in Pink*. I was beyond moved when Duckie said to Andie, "This is a really volcanic ensemble you're wearing, it's really marvelous!" I wanted to be her so badly. I had the naturally red hair and everything. I desperately wanted to make pretty clothes out of thrift-shop rejects and date rich, Brat Pack boys from the right side of the tracks who wore cream-colored linen suits to school. Why couldn't that be me?

I got a little sidetracked from my dream and got married and had kids instead, but in 2000, I went back to school and earned a second bachelor's degree, in fashion design, hoping to embark on a career as a costume designer for film and television in the very un-Hollywoodlike city of Portland, Oregon. Oddly, I made it happen. Granted, I don't work on big, expensive studio movies. I've worked on a few really bad independent films that went straight to video, but mostly I work on television commercials. And I'm not really a costume designer. I'm a wardrobe stylist, but close enough. After graduation, I landed at a small production company producing national commercials for what used to be Will Vinton Studios — think dancing California Raisins and talking M&M's. No, I did not dress raisins or candy; we also did spots for Wrigley's, Trident, and Hostess that had real actors in them.

I've styled the costumes for over a hundred commercials, including national spots for Toyota, Nike, Nickelodeon, and Blockbuster. I don't watch TV (because I hate the commercials), but you've probably seen some of mine. I specialize in dressing soccer moms. The kids aren't the only ones wearing a uniform. At least in TV land, soccer moms wear a blue, button-front, collared shirt with long sleeves (very neatly rolled up by yours truly) worn untucked over slightly faded jeans with barely worn tennis shoes. Sometimes I go a little crazy and layer the blue outer shirt with a pale yellow T-shirt underneath to polish off the look. Clearly, the wardrobe on a typical commercial isn't all that exciting, but every once in a while, I travel to Los Angeles for something a little more fabulous, like the network image campaigns. You've seen them — those promo spots on TV with stars dressed in fancy designer clothing with their hands on their hips looking sultry or tough depending on the character they play. I've done quite a few of those, for *House*, *Veronica Mars*, *Hell's Kitchen*, and other shows. The money sucks, but the food is awesome, and the clothes are unreal and a true pleasure to shop for on Rodeo Drive and at Neiman's of Beverly Hills. Designer denim is my personal addiction.

For me, wardrobe has been a great motivator for maintaining

my weight. I look forward to getting dressed and putting on my favorite jeans, a fitted vintage blouse, and a badass pair of boots. And when those jeans feel a little snug, I rein it back in. I see nothing wrong with a little vanity if it keeps you slender and trim. My so-called vanity has helped to prevent knee, hip, and back problems that many people my age suffer from and began to experience in their twenties and thirties often due to simply carrying around excess weight. I have never seen a chiropractor, a podiatrist, or an orthopedic physician, and I plan to keep it that way for as long as possible. Having said that, I would like to stress that overall health and not actual weight is where you should place your emphasis. That means that getting adequate exercise is a critical component to lifelong wellness (more on this in Item #13). Being slender and unfit is not what I would characterize as *healthy*. My love of fashion helps keep me on track, but what you'll find in this book is a "whole-body" approach to being healthy.

THE DENIM DIARY

Due to a flight cancellation en route to a family holiday, I took an unplanned six-hour drive from Dallas to the Texas Panhandle. It was my first trip to Texas. Along the way, I saw numerous billboards for seventy-two-ounce steaks and a mind-blowing number of obese people. The road trip ended in Amarillo, where I stayed with friends and family. I couldn't help but notice that nine out of ten restaurants were fast-food establishments with lines going around the block. A place called The Donut Stop (I'm fairly certain I counted seven of them) was a far more common sighting than a gym or anyone running or even walking. While visiting a store called Sheplers in search of the perfect pair of Wranglers, I came across a pair of jeans so large that I jokingly said to my friend that even the denim needed to go on a diet.

The lunch scene at the Cracker Barrel restaurant that same day made my jaw drop. I saw overflowing platefuls of greasy, fried, gravy-laden food being zealously devoured by patrons with bellies so large that they could barely reach the meal in front of them. What I saw was Fat America. For the rest of the afternoon, I took a lengthy but restless nap. Immediately upon waking up, I grabbed from my suitcase a blank journal that I'd purchased at the airport in Portland. Looking back, I think the fact that I bought a journal is more than a little odd because I've never journaled a day in my life. Back in high school, I kept a record of boys I kissed and what I was wearing at the time, but that's as extensive as my diary-keeping efforts went. My brain was now on serious overdrive, and without a moment's hesitation, I began to write the first draft of this manuscript. Within five days, it was finished and *The Denim Diet* was born. As you will discover later, it has actually been swirling around in my head for over twenty years; it just took a Texas-size kick in the ass for me to get pen to paper.

As I mentioned, I live in Portland, Oregon, and work in the film and television business. I'm surrounded by either ultraskinny, neurotic actresses or vegan, eco-centric, outdoor-sports enthusiasts who bike to work, snowboard all winter, windsurf all summer, and march the streets of Portland to prevent the likes of Wal-Mart and Target from taking hold within the urban growth boundary. Most assuredly, there are Portlanders who could stand to lose a few pounds, but I had to leave home to be reminded of just how fat this country really is. Texas was the birthplace of my moment of inspiration, but I in no way want to offend the kind folks that call it home. Admittedly, I'm off to an irreverent start, but the people I met there were incredibly hospitable and welcoming, and I am grateful for my time there. I assure you, I'll lighten up. Let's all lighten up.

I've had my share of years when I struggled with my weight. Twenty-two years ago, my jeans were six sizes larger than they are today, and I was diagnosed with high blood pressure and put on medication. We're all in this together. With 142 million overweight or obese adult Americans, we as a society clearly do not understand how to eat healthily. Included in that figure are Americans with medical conditions such as thyroid disorders and other debilitating diseases that cause them to gain weight beyond their control. The comments and guidance in this book are not directed at those individuals, and I have the greatest sympathy for their health struggles. This book is for everyone else included in that staggering number — the overweight, obese, and morbidly obese people whose choices and habits have made us the fattest country in the world.

I believe we're in this predicament because many Americans don't know the basics of healthy eating or how to have a positive relationship with food. And that's okay, because I do and I'm going to share what I know with you — the simple habits that helped me lose weight and keep it off for over twenty years without yo-yo dieting or starving myself. In the same way that many people struggle with diet and weight loss, I used to struggle with office organization — we all have weak areas, and that was one of mine. Maybe it should have been completely obvious to me how to keep my office organized, but until I had someone with a passion and an expertise in office organization train me on new habits and show me how to simplify my system, I kept failing over and over. I don't go digging through my drawers to find a receipt anymore — mainly because the office tyrant took away my drawers, but also because I've developed new habits that prevent me from emptying my pockets and purse into a giant black hole. I knew my old system was inefficient and causing me a great deal of stress at tax time, but I wasn't able to develop another system on my own that worked. Expert advice helped me change that. I hope that in a similar way, my insights into healthy eating will help you gain control of your weight. What I know is an easy and effortless solution to being fat, and I've spent twenty years sharing my simple philosophy with friends, family, a few Hollywood actors, and anyone else who would listen. I know how to lose the fat, keep it off, have tons of energy, eat plenty of food, do better by Mother Earth, and look and feel like the picture of health. What I'm about to share with you has worked flawlessly for me through postpregnancy, motherhood, divorce, turning forty, and countless dinner parties, weddings, Sunday brunches, and family vacations.

Before Joe, my literary agent, agreed to take me on as a

client, he asked me a very important and fair question and one I hadn't given much thought to. He asked, "Who are you, Kami, and why are *you* writing this book?" He was essentially saying, You're no expert, you're not a doctor, you're not a dietician — why should anyone listen to you? I joke and say I have a PhD (Pretty Hot in Denim), but who I am is *you*. I'm a regular person who figured out long ago how to live my life in a healthy way and by doing so has managed to maintain an ideal, healthy body weight, easily and effortlessly. That's the real secret: You don't need to be a doctor or a registered dietician to figure it out. You can be you — just a regular person who wants to have a healthy, slim body that lasts for as long as possible. Don't get me wrong — healthcare providers are an absolute necessity. Even though I don't understand half of what they tell me, I call on them regularly. I also do my own research and read every available word about health and wellness and then apply my own experience, logic, and what my body tells me. Sometimes I get my facts, figures, and information from what I call the *Journal of Commonsense Eating*, an imaginary publication that I've been compiling in my head for the past twenty or so years. Now, in my very regular-person voice, I'm going to pass on to you all that I know and have learned, in the hope that you can benefit from my simple, no-nonsense approach to eating well to create a healthy, slim, and hopefully pain-free, disease-free, and long-lasting body. As a major bonus, if you follow what I've presented here, you will not only get into your dream pair of jeans; you will become a better steward of the

Earth as a natural consequence of the habits, activities, and choices you're making.

True to my Oregon roots, the philosophy in this book ties in beautifully with being and thinking green. You'll learn how to easily and effortlessly lose weight, but in doing so, you'll be able to feel good about lessening your impact on Earth's energy and resources. Not that I wouldn't, but I'm not jumping on the eco-bandwagon. My parents are two of the bandleaders. My mom designs and builds solar homes and is a pioneer of the green building movement. She's practiced organic gardening since the seventies (long before it was popular), and I grew up living in her beautiful solar homes. My dad is currently working to install a thousand-acre wind farm on Montana land he inherited from his homesteading grandmother. Collectively, they harvest their own electricity through their "goal net zero" floating home (and sell the surplus to neighbors through the utility company), drive hybrids, grow organic vegetables and herbs on their rooftop garden, and open their home for solar and green tours on weekends. Mom and Dad are constantly in the news, most recently in a feature article in *Wired* magazine, and a documentary filmmaker is highlighting their efforts on his upcoming project. (No, it's not Al Gore. It is a very talented someone, but the parents have given me a gag order, and I'm still somewhat of an obedient child.) I've been schooled on green — ironically, by the Grays. My parents have taught me that being lean works brilliantly with being green.

FRENCH FRIES, FRITOS,
AND THE FRESHMAN FIFTEEN

When it came to food, I used to get away with a lot. Flash back to twenty-eight years ago (I'm trying to make my story more dramatic just in case Ron Howard wants to make my book into a movie) when I was a freshman in high school and we had to count our daily calories as part of a health class assignment. Mine added up to four thousand calories a day on average. At the time, I thought that had to be fairly close to the recommended daily target since there wasn't an ounce of fat on me.

Four years later, after my first semester at Arizona State University, that definitely wasn't the case. The Sun Devils were a bunch of good-looking rich kids (many from Southern California) who had performed only slightly above average in high school and liked to party. By December, I was fat and I was a total misfit. Apparently, if you grew up in "SoCal," you had some special gene that prevented you from getting fat. I sure didn't have it. I came from Oregon, and the only other girl in my sorority to get fat like me was from Idaho. She became my best friend. Together we were Ore-Ida, and boy did we eat a lot of French fries.

When I went home for winter vacation, I heard comments like "They must not require a P.E. class at your school" and "Looks like you're not there for an MRS degree, like your dad said." That doesn't stand for "Masters of Really Skinny." That means my dad thought I went to college to find myself a husband

and become somebody's Mrs. The unsolicited commentary that irked me the most came from my uncle Jim: "Back in my day, it was the freshman fifteen. Did that go up with college tuition?" That's a good one, Uncle Jim — a real knee-slapper! For those of you who don't know, "freshman fifteen" refers to the number of pounds a typical college frosh can expect to gain. I was well beyond that, and worse, I mistakenly thought I was loved and adored unconditionally. Deep down I knew my family still loved me, but I was laying on the self-pity as thick as the butter and fake maple syrup on my Belgian waffles.

So I was a little round. A little doughy — kind of like a Belgian waffle, proving that you are, in fact, what you eat. I wasn't thrilled about it, but I thought it was beyond my control. I didn't attribute it to all the fattening food I was eating: Flakey Jake's fried chicken sandwiches on giant white buns grilled with mystery grease, French fries drenched in thick orange cheddar-cheese sauce, and family-size bowls of fro-yo (aka frozen yogurt) with crumbled Heath bar topping. Without question, the increase in partying didn't help matters, but it never dawned on me that my poor eating habits had finally caught up with me — habits like hitting the vending machines (endearingly referred to as Vendoland by me and my friends) in the dorm hall at midnight and eating as much junk food as I could afford with my saved-up laundry quarters. This usually meant I couldn't wash my clothes that week, but they were getting too snug anyway. That didn't stop me from being first in line when the dorm cafeteria served Fritos Con Carne every Wednesday night.

INTRODUCTION

When I wasn't eating at Vendoland, a sorority sister from South Dakota was my dining companion on many occasions. I'll call her Miss South Dakota, since she could easily have been a beauty pageant winner. Miss South Dakota was thin. Not sickeningly thin. She looked amazing and was so damn pleasant and happy all the time. Looking back, I'm sure I completely grossed her out by what I ate, how much of it I ate, and how quickly I ate it. Wherever you are, Miss South Dakota, I sincerely apologize.

When Miss South Dakota went to Flakey Jake's, she ordered a plain turkey patty. All the extras come on the side at Flakey's. She would load her "base" up with steamed broccoli, pinto beans, corn, garbanzo beans, tomatoes, and salsa. She made a giant mound of food. No bun. No mayonnaise. No melted cheese. I thought it was really weird and that maybe Miss South Dakota had some kind of rare disorder and couldn't eat normal, tasty food. I was just too polite to ask her about it. Actually, that's a lie — I was too busy licking my fingers and stuffing my fat face with grease and lard.

I've since learned that sweatpants make you look a lot fatter than a pair of jeans that are the right size for you, but back then, when it became abundantly clear that I would be dressing myself in only elastic-waisted shorts and sweatpants and tying a sweatshirt around my waist to cover my ever-expanding ass, the guy I was dating broke up with me. He said he just wanted to hang with the fellas and not have a girlfriend. Within a week, he was dating a superskinny sorority sister of mine from Hawaii who later became a swimsuit model.

By the end of my freshman year, I had gained some serious weight. Not only did I now have a big ass and an almost perfectly round face; my mood was becoming quite foul. I was also beginning to have trouble sleeping because it was uncomfortable to snooze on my stomach. After finals, I went back home to Oregon with my tail between my chubby legs. I spent the entire summer vacation obsessed with losing the weight. I did aerobics seven days a week (yes, I wore a thong leotard) and completely starved myself. I lost the weight, went back to school, and promptly got the boyfriend back. But by midterms, I had gained it all back — plus several pounds. The boyfriend hung in there with me, sweatpants and all, likely because his bad eating habits had finally caught up with him. With his expanding midsection came his own affinity for elastic-waisted attire, and as luck would have it, he didn't find me quite so unattractive this time around.

At the insistence of my boyfriend, who was growing tired of paying for all our gluttonous meals, I got a job as a hostess at the Radisson Resort Restaurant in Scottsdale, Arizona. Thanks to the Carl's Jr. Super Stars with cheese that I chowed down each day during my commute to work, I was at my absolute fattest. We had to dress in "nicer" clothes at the Radisson, meaning no college tank tops or sweatpants. I was forced to purchase a few items that would be presentable for work. My roommate was from Las Vegas, just shy of six feet, and a beanpole, which I thought was really odd. Not the beanpole part; the Las Vegas part — I didn't realize until I met her that you could *be* from Las Vegas. I thought people only visited her hometown to see the absolute worst of America and eat steak dinners for $4.99. Regardless of my confusion, borrowing her clothes was not really an option . . . except this one very desperate time.

I had nothing to wear. My clothes were in a massive pile, clean mixed with dirty, lying at the bottom of my luxurious two-foot-wide closet. My roomie, who wasn't home, had her clothes arranged all nicely and neatly. (Is it just me, or are skinny girls more organized?) I spotted a short black-and-white-print cotton skirt with an elastic waist in her closet. Score! It was really tight, but thanks to a slit up the back, I managed to squeeze my way into it. To camouflage my butt (and the fact that I was wearing a skirt that was four sizes too small for me), I found a black oversize blouse in my pile and pinned a sparkly rhinestone brooch at the neck (just like Molly Ringwald did in the movie).

About halfway through my shift, as I bent down to pick up a customer's napkin that had fallen on the floor, one of the waitresses, who for some reason hated my guts ('course, I kind of hated me too) said, "Your slit is so high, I can see your underwear." Awesome. I knew she was lying because I hadn't been able to find any clean underwear (thank God it was the eighties and I had worn panty hose), but the slit on the skirt had split all the way up my backside. This was a serious low point. I grabbed my purse, walked out the door of the restaurant and of the hotel, got into my crappy peach-colored Datsun B210, and sobbed all the way home. My eyes were so puffy that my roommate instantly forgave me for stealing and ruining her skirt.

Adding insult to injury, she said it was too big for her and that I could have it. Oh boy!

I spent the next two years in college fat and getting increasingly fatter. In the back of my mind, though, I never stopped thinking about Miss South Dakota's big mound of protein and vegetables. I don't remember discussing food or diet with her, but I guess subconsciously I had been taking notes. Somewhere in the middle of my junior year, I had a revelation. Miss South Dakota was a genius! *She ate a lot of food.* She was never hungry and was always in a great mood. She had lots of energy and looked fabulous. She ate the right food. She saw food as fuel. I needed to change the way I thought about food. Miss South Dakota made the right choices, and I made the wrong choices. *What I eat is a choice!* This was huge.

So I changed my mind. I changed my thinking. I had been thinking myself fat, and now I would think myself thin. Miss South Dakota was my inspiration, but I also had been raised by a mom who, for the most part, valued "real" food. I just thought it tasted kind of gross. The entire reason I had babysat as an adolescent was to eat food at other people's houses: Kraft Macaroni and Cheese, Swanson TV dinners, Cap'n Crunch cereal, and Popsicles (real, packaged ones — not the kind that Mom made by mixing and freezing orange juice and grape juice, which resulted in a frozen gray mass that appeared to have lint stuck in it). It was now time to embrace the kind of real food I had done my best to avoid as a skinny kid.

INTRODUCTION

THE LEAN SIXTEEN

After my colossal epiphany, I slowly retrained myself and developed new habits — starting with how I look at food. My new attitude: Food is a beautiful thing. It replenishes me and restores me. It makes me strong and healthy. It revs me up and keeps me going. Food is fuel, and it works for me and serves me. Once I clearly saw the simplicity and perfection in seeing food as fuel, the fat disappeared and, with the exception of two wonderful nine-month periods of pregnancy, has stayed off for over two decades. As I mentioned earlier, I am not a dietician and I am not a doctor (although I do dress them on TV), and this book is not another "diet" book. I have a confession to make. I know it's in the title to this book, but I think the word *diet* sucks. It implies that for a temporary period of time, your eating habits will need to change dramatically in order for you to achieve weight loss. Instead of dictating a diet, I'm going to introduce you to sixteen simple habits to easily and effortlessly practice and develop so you don't have to think about how great it would be to lose weight and keep it off; you'll be living it, one simple habit at a time. I call these sixteen simple habits "the List." The List is not a new fad diet. As a wardrobe stylist and, worse, a product of the eighties, I can tell you all about fads and the latest trends. In three words, *they don't last*. The List, on the other hand, is for the rest of your life.

You'll get plenty of specific guidance and learn my philosophy of good eating and living, but it all starts with changing the way you think about food. It's not complicated. Food is either on the List or not on the List. Items that are on the List are habits to make, and items that are not on the List are habits to break. By the time you've finished reading this book, you'll get it. Some may get it well before that. How awesome would it be to develop sixteen simple habits and, in doing so, lose weight and keep it that way forever?

The List is simple, just like my vocabulary. We've come to rely on fad diets, pills, surgery, and even mail-order food as the answers to fat. I tried some stupid stuff myself and have learned that finding the quick fix is not the answer. Fake, "lite," diet, fat-free food is not the answer. Starving yourself is so not the answer. The solution is far easier and healthier, and it lasts forever. What you need is good food that fuels your body — beautiful, wonderful, perfect, real food — not processed, bleached, and refined food with nasty chemicals and fillers in it. Your body will respond by shedding the layers of fat, giving you abundant energy, providing you with a vehicle for a longer, healthier life, and looking like the picture of well-being on the inside and out. Sound good?

If what you truly want for yourself is a healthy, slim body, become a better decision maker. I have found that, surprisingly, it's not about discipline. It's about making good decisions. And these are easy decisions to make — split-second, yes-or-no decisions. Nothing too challenging like deciding whether you should end your dead-end relationship or whether to take the kids to Hawaii or Mexico for spring break (neither — hire Grandma or a babysitter, leave the kids at home, and go to

Italy). Just yes or no. Soon you will be developing new habits
— lifelong habits that you will stick to easily and effortlessly.

I'm not fat, but I'm not skin and bones either. I've got a few
curves. Being ultraskinny grosses me out. (You may have noticed
that I use the word *gross* a lot. Keep in mind that I went to college at the biggest party school in the nation, where our motto
was "C = B.A." and we frequently used words like *gross* on term
papers. If we really wanted to impress our professors, we used
supergross, but we had to use it sparingly. Plus, I just really like
the word. I think it's grossly underrated. Too cheesy? We'll be
discussing cheese later, so let's not get off topic.) The bodies of
Hollywood stars are pretty much the size we all were in sixth or
seventh grade. I'm not just talking about the women here. Moreover, actors need a lot of reassurance that they have zero body
fat. Part of my job as a wardrobe stylist is to keep the actors
happy. Not exactly a small order, since many are majorly inse-
cure, and most are in dire need of a proper meal but would prefer to bite my head off instead. I had to shop for one teeny-tiny
twenty-eight-year-old (so she says) actress in the children's
department. As exciting as it's been to dress stars like Kristen
Bell, Jenny McCarthy, Shannen Doherty, Hugh Laurie, Taye
Diggs, Michael Michele, John Corbett, Amy Smart, Patty Duke,
and Sean Astin, being in this industry has made me acutely
aware of how important it is not to worship what you see in
tabloid magazines. It's not real and it's not really possible, at least
not for very long. I have been thinner than I am today, but even
a five-pound loss zaps my energy and obliterates my curves, and
the good plumpness on my face completely disappears. I'm

forty-one as I'm writing this, and when my ass starts to shrink, my face shrivels up right along with it. High-definition TV is not your friend, Hollywood actors! Your friend is a peanut butter and jelly sandwich (get excited — PB&Js, slightly modified, are on the List).

I know what my best weight is. I know because it pretty much stays there without much effort. In their weekly newspaper column, "The YOU Docs," Mehmet Oz, MD, and Michael Roizen, MD, suggest looking at your high school yearbook. They say that your body was at its most metabolically efficient at that time, and those yearbook photos "provide a ballpark idea of where you want your body to be today." (Note: that's your *body*, not your hairstyle or eye-shadow color.) Thanks to gravity and having children, things have shifted downward, but my Levi's 501s from high school would still fit me today. (My old bikini? Not so much — not even in a ballpark sort of way.) Another good way to determine your ideal, healthy weight is to calculate your BMI, or body mass index. The BMI measures the ratio between height and weight. These are just guidelines, but a BMI between 18.5 and 24.9 indicates a normal, healthy weight. To determine your BMI, divide your weight in pounds by your height in inches. Then divide the answer by your height in inches. Multiply the answer by 703. I'm severely math challenged (I tested into Level 087 Math when I arrived at college, and college courses start with a number 1), so I use a calculator and even mess that up half the time. Fortunately, the Department of Health and Human Services has a handy BMI calculator online at www.nhlbisupport.com/bmi.

BMI CATEGORIES:
UNDERWEIGHT = less than 18.5
NORMAL WEIGHT = 18.5–24.9
OVERWEIGHT = 25–29.9
OBESE = 30 or greater

The BMI doesn't tell the whole story, though. Normal-weight people can still be obese. Obesity is an excess of fat, not of weight. Come again? A person with a healthy weight can have a high percentage of body fat — "high" meaning 30 percent or more — and still be in the normal BMI range. Most fitness centers have machines that measure body fat through a technique called Bioimpedance. Sounds a little scary, but it's a quick and painless technique that looks at body composition using an electrical current. There are other devices, like calipers, that measure body fat as well. Why should you care? Because according to a Mayo Clinic study led by cardiologist Francisco Lopez-Jimenez, MD, excessive body fat can lead to high blood pressure, abnormal cholesterol levels, and insulin resistance and puts you at an increased risk for type 2 diabetes. That means that, as I suggested earlier, along with changing your eating habits, it's time to get some exercise. But not to worry — when you follow the List, you should have plenty of energy for a half-hour walk. And if not, you can do as the YOU Docs, Dr. Oz and Dr. Roizen, suggest: break it up into ten-minute walks until you have the strength and stamina for the full thirty minutes. If you're already incorporating regular exercise into your weekly routine, it might still be a good idea to get your percentage of body fat checked, if for no other reason than to give yourself a giant pat on the back. You deserve it. (And I'll talk more about exercise in Item #13.)

As you develop new habits and change the way you look at food, make sure you listen to your body. You should communicate any concerns to your doctor. I'm not saying this because I have to. I've had the same doctor since I was nine years old. Anyone who knows me will tell you I see my doctor regularly. My friends will say it's because I'm a hypochondriac, but I would argue that it's because I have a zest for life and want to make sure that I'm the healthiest I can be. (Plus, my doctor is kind of handsome. I say that even though I saw him at Home Depot once and he couldn't remember my name — after thirty-two years. That kind of sucked.) In any case, you might want to consult your doctor and make sure you don't have any health issues before you make any significant dietary changes.

People who know me also know that I eat a ton of food. My plate at dinner usually has the most on it. Newcomers to our family gatherings often stare and make comments about how much I can "put away." It is *what* I eat that makes all the difference. I have trained myself, and you can too. When I'm hungry, I don't think about what sounds delicious or what would taste amazing; I think about what would quickly satiate me and fuel my body, and I make sure I have plenty of things on hand that will do the job. I call this "purposeful eating" because everything I put into my body, I eat on purpose. You will learn to tweak your current eating habits as opposed to giving up your favorite foods. On the List, you can still have your coffee, dairy, meat, and wine, just in a more conscientious and healthful way.

My relationship with food requires no willpower. Either foods are on the List or they aren't. It's *yes* or *no*, and I've trained myself to make a habit of eating only *yes* foods. And I've changed the way I think about those foods; I see them as fuel that makes my body strong, efficient, energetic, and satisfied, with very little excess fat. I no longer even have to *try* to limit myself to the *yes* foods; I just do it. When you start following the List, remember what Jedi Master Yoda said: "Try not. Do... or do not. There is no try." (Yes, I'm aware that Yoda is a petite, fictional character from a space movie series. But he was pretty wise. And it's not like I said, "May the force be with you" ...although I'm secretly hoping it is.) You can do this. You can lose the fat and be a healthier, stronger, and slimmer you.

Also, realize that each step is as important as the next. While you are changing your old habits and practicing new ones, celebrate each step you make toward a better you. You can change your mind and the decisions you make. As Byron Katie, one of the great transformational speakers of our time, says, "There are no physical problems — only mental ones." For your body to be healthy, your mind needs to think healthy.

What does it mean to be healthy? Being at your ideal weight is only one aspect of good health. Following the List will help you be the picture of health on the inside too — where it matters the most. Eating well can help guard against disease, cancer, and a multitude of other ailments as well as improve your energy and mental health. Increased longevity is another natural by-product of making good dietary choices.

And let's not overlook planetary health. Being slim and trim won't get us too far if we don't have a healthy environment to exist in. The List helps you to become slimmer and healthier while you simultaneously minimize the impact you make on Earth's energy and resources.

The List is a "good is good enough" philosophy, as opposed to a hard-core set of rules, which could lead to obsessive behavior and make us feel like failures. I learned the phrase "good is good enough" many years ago, when I was working through some parenting issues with a therapist. She was trying to help me overcome my need to be Supermom to my children because it created feelings of guilt and failure rather than satisfaction and enjoyment. The same idea applies here. For many of us, overly restrictive rules, diets, and striving for perfection feel overwhelming and set us up for repeated failure — and it's boring! I'm convinced that the majority of us want the same thing: to live a long, healthy life and to leave the Earth in the best condition possible for our children, grandchildren, and future generations. So be good, and sometimes even be great — and try your utmost to avoid being destructive and causing harm to your body, to fellow humans, or to our planet. Even if you feel like some of the guidance I suggest in this book doesn't work for you, skip to the next habit or come back to that one when you feel ready and willing. I can tell you that I live by all of them, and I don't have to worry about my weight. For me that's important because I've got a closet full of jeans to fit into. But rather than feeling overwhelmed by the List, find what makes sense to you. Take your time, try out new things, and let new ideas, concepts, and actions take root so they can blossom into habits.

Some people may find my attitude too lenient, complacent, or compromising. I would say, *Lighten up!* I would also say that it's all the little good things we do over long periods of time that add up to real, measurable achievement. Some people have shared with me that their body is so out of control and so far gone and the planet is such a mess that they feel helpless; they ask what they can do to reverse the situation and create real change. Little things, that's what! This book is about these little things — these little good things that can make a world of difference toward having a healthier body and a healthier planet.

I've read many self-help books on a wide array of topics. The ones that have appealed to me the most are those that got up close and personal. Self-help books that only teach and preach bore me silly after a few chapters. They also make me feel incapable of establishing a connection with the author or a sense of confidence in their advice or whether or not it could work for me. Nor do I appreciate being lectured at or badgered with heavy-handed tactics and overly technical language. So I've tried to create a book that's more intimate, sensible, and understanding. Just like you, I'm a real person. I'm happy to share my own experiences, issues, triumphs, and setbacks. I don't stop there, though. Oh no; I share other people's stories as well. With the exception of my sister's, whom I repeatedly throw under the bus, I don't divulge any names because I didn't *exactly* get anyone's permission. Some of these stories are humorous, a few are inspirational, others provide living examples of weight-loss success, and one is a dramatic life lesson in what *not* to do. I refer to these stories as "Food for Thought," and they are designed to entertain, encourage, and motivate you but, more important, to bring us together. That's not to say there isn't specific guidance and plenty of good, solid information in each and every chapter. I also provide a complete grocery list to get you started by stocking your refrigerator and pantry with foods on the List. Thirty-one recipes are included in the back of the book as well, ranging from soups and salads to homemade breads. And since I'm a wardrobe stylist, it would be a shame to miss an opportunity to share with you my top ten tips for dressing to look slimmer. They're also toward the end of the book, along with a handy four-page summary of the List for those times when you need a quick refresher on all the great habits you will soon be developing.

The List gives you sixteen simple habits to easily and effortlessly practice and develop: a plan with just enough why and plenty of how in a "let's tackle one thing at a time, and it's all interrelated and not at all complicated" type of approach with some personal stories to keep you entertained and maintain your enthusiasm along the way. Take pleasure in taking this time for yourself and taking better care of you!

SODA POP, GUMMY BEARS, AND YOUR SWEET TOOTH

Slimming Alternatives to High Fructose Corn Syrup, Sugar, and Artificial Sweeteners

We are what we repeatedly do.
Excellence is therefore not an act, but a habit.
— Aristotle

WITH THE EXCEPTION OF ILLEGAL DRUGS and cigarettes, soda (or soft drinks or pop or whatever you call it) is the single stupidest thing that we put into our bodies. Before I completely go off on diet soda, let's talk about the big fat problem called *high fructose corn syrup* (HFCS). This is likely the sweetener that is in your "sugary" soda drink and in your gummy bears and in a frightening number of other things that Americans eat and drink regularly. It's bad news. It's big fat bad news.

A little common sense tells me that this stuff is a huge player in the obesity epidemic. Here's a strange coincidence: Obesity in America spiked in the 1980s and has continued to rise. The 1980s were when the world's two largest soda companies introduced high fructose corn syrup in their products. By the

1990s, high fructose corn syrup was used in hundreds of grocery store items. (In case you're wondering, yes, I see the irony, or rather the hypocrisy, in the fact that in my commercial work, I've helped peddle a bunch of products that contain high fructose corn syrup!)

The *American Journal of Clinical Nutrition* has published several studies on the effects of high fructose corn syrup on the body. In an editorial on the journal's website, George A. Bray writes, "The intake of soft drinks containing high-fructose corn syrup (HFCS) or sucrose has risen in parallel with the epidemic of obesity, which suggests a relation." An article titled "What's Worse Than Sugar?" quotes Richard Anderson, a scientist at the federal Human Nutrition Research Center, as saying, "I think it's a huge problem. High-fructose corn syrup is metabolized differently than other sugars, and it has a different effect on health." Kim Severson, a staff writer for the *San Francisco Chronicle*, also chimes in about the situation, saying, "The theory goes like this: The body processes the fructose in high fructose corn syrup differently than it does old-fashioned cane or beet sugar, which in turn alters the way metabolic-regulating hormones function. It also forces the liver to kick more fat out into the bloodstream. The end result is that our bodies are essentially tricked into wanting to eat more and at the same time, we are storing more fat."

Although there are scores of articles that identify HFCS as the bad guy, there are at least as many that say the opposite. The American Medical Association announced, "after examining the evidence, that high fructose corn syrup doesn't appear to contribute more to obesity than other sweeteners but called for further research into its long-term effects." Have you noticed that whenever corporate America stands to lose big dollars, we get oodles of conflicting evidence and research? This is, not surprisingly, the case with high fructose corn syrup.

That doesn't make a lick of difference to me. Despite the inconclusive research, here's what I've managed to scrape together: Regular sugar (or glucose) is processed in your cells and then metabolized by your liver in an orderly fashion. Your liver has plenty of information to decide what to do with those glucose molecules: store them as glycogen, use them for energy, or, if you've already got plenty stored up and don't seem to be expending much energy (exercising), use them for fat storage. HFCS goes on a different journey. It isn't processed in your cells and takes a more direct route to your liver. When it arrives, since it hasn't been processed in your cells, your liver is lacking vital information that helps it determine what to do next, so it does what is easiest — throws it into fat storage. Enzymes are released that instruct your body to store the fructose molecules as fat — meaning it isn't available to be converted to energy that your body can use or burn off.

That's outstanding news if you like belly fat. People read the fat-free labeling on products that are mostly HFCS and think they're eating diet food, but in reality, when HFCS enters your body, it acts more like fat than sugar does. Ever wonder why you can eat handfuls of fat-free, "diet" food or drink multiple cans of soda? Because of the way HFCS is metabolized in your body, it's unlikely to stimulate insulin production, which is what sends a signal to your brain that you're full and satiated. And so you keep on eating — or drinking, in the case of soda pop.

The United States Department of Agriculture says that the average American consumes sixty pounds of HFCS per year. That amount could easily translate into twenty, thirty, or even forty pounds of weight gain — of fat. Guess how much we were consuming in 1970? A half a pound per year. Guess when we started becoming the fattest nation on the planet? In the 1980s, when, coincidentally, HFCS took over as the new, cheap sweetener of choice in Coke, Pepsi, and scads of other products. What if you didn't eat any foods containing HFCS for the following year (and then for the rest of your life) and lost that extra fat instead? Wouldn't that be awesome?

The saddest part about the common use of HFCS is what it has done to our nation's children. I was at a dinner party recently and the couple's adorable little kids were running around, playing, and entertaining us. They were also eating Popsicles one after the other and drinking soda pop when thirsty. The oldest daughter had little stick legs and arms but a large protruding belly for her size. Believe me, I put away my share of Popsicles and soda pop as a kid, but I grew up before corn was refined into a sweetener and added to everything from ketchup to pancake syrup. We ate pure cane sugar. My mouth is littered with dental fillings to prove it. Today's youth may also spend more time using computers and doing other sedentary activities than some of us did as kids, and there are undeniably other contributors to childhood obesity, but we can easily eliminate this one major obstacle to maintaining a healthy body weight — for our children and for ourselves.

Think you're not consuming much HFCS? Read your labels carefully because there are tons of products that contain it. Don't be fooled by products that are labeled as "100% natural" or "all natural," such as many Snapple beverages and Newman's Own Lemonade and Limeade. As of this writing, the FDA has no definition for these terms (although a petition is reportedly in the works), so food manufacturers are "naturally" free and loose with them. In addition to soda, Popsicles, ketchup, and pancake syrup, products containing HFCS include sports and energy drinks, sweetened tea beverages, jelly, frozen entrées, pasta sauce, barbecue sauce, flavored mustard, chocolate syrup, salad dressing, juice boxes, so-called fruit drinks, ice cream, sandwich bread, and most candy.

The two that shocked me the most are chocolate syrup and kid's juice boxes. Check out the label on a bottle of Hershey's Chocolate Syrup. When you read labels, it's important to realize that ingredients are listed in order of predominance, with the ingredient used in the highest amount first, followed by other ingredients in descending order. Cocoa is listed as the fifth ingredient in Hershey's Syrup, after HFCS, corn syrup, water, and sugar. That means that there is a greater amount of all four of those items than actual cocoa. Capri Sun Orange "juice drink," which is targeted to kids, contains more water and HFCS than actual juice. Fast food contains a lot of HFCS too. Go to www.foodfacts.info/high-fructose-corn-syrup.shtml to see the staggering list of fast-food menu items that contain the awful stuff.

The corn refiners and beverage companies and plenty of others that make the big bucks off this stuff will do their best to convince you that HFCS is a natural part of a healthy diet. One of my workshop students asked me recently how I sort out all the conflicting research and evidence that we are constantly bombarded with concerning food products and ingredients like HFCS. I told her I don't. I keep it simple and don't pay any attention to the hype. I eat foods that existed long before I was here. Does it surprise me that Pepsi helped fund the latest "research" on HFCS and claims that it's really no different from regular white, refined sugar? Not at all. I disagree whole-heartedly, but it doesn't matter to me whatsoever, because: 1) I avoid refined food, including white sugar; and 2) common sense tells me to steer clear of ingredients that are comprised of four words strung together. To me, that sounds complicated, man-ufactured, fake, and toxic. The foods I eat don't contain ingre-dients that sound like laboratory-created chemicals. I also avoid foods that have an endless list of ingredients. Giant food manu-facturers have taken the food out of our food and replaced it with chemicals, preservatives, and poison that make us fatter and fatter and full of disease and cancer, and they've packaged our food in a way that creates truckloads of waste and ensures our de-pendence on nonrenewable resources like oil. I say, trust your common sense, your instincts, and your ever-expanding gut.

And speaking of consumables that create a larger waistline,

ITEM #1: YOUR SWEET TOOTH

for those of you who drink the Jones brand of designer sodas, which recently switched from HFCS to pure cane sugar, you're not off the hook, either (even though their bottle designs are clever and beyond cool). Neither are the rest of you who are consuming beverages or processed foods containing cane sugar or beet sugar. These two processed sugars are derived from different plants, but food labels may or may not indicate which is included. Since beet sugar is cheaper to process, there's a good chance your processed or packaged foods contain beet sugar as opposed to cane. It's all the same to me. If I were you, I would stay away from both of them. Sugar can lead to tooth decay and an imbalance in insulin levels, but it can also tack on a bunch of empty calories to your daily intake, which in turn can make you fat. Sugar adds calories but nothing in the way of nutrition. How many calories? I'm really glad you asked. You ready? Each bottle of Jones root beer, for example, has 180 calories and contains about ten teaspoons of sugar. Can you imagine putting that much sugar in your cup of coffee? Give or take a few teaspoons, the list below can be applied to other brands as well. I know some of you don't stop at just one bottle or can a day, so here's a handy guide of approximately how much sugar and how many calories you're consuming with every twelve-ounce bottle:

ONE SODA: 10 teaspoons of sugar and 180 calories
TWO SODAS: 20 teaspoons of sugar and 360 calories
THREE SODAS: 30 teaspoons of sugar and 540 calories
FOUR SODAS: 40 teaspoons of sugar and 720 calories

FIVE SODAS: 50 teaspoons of sugar and 900 calories
SIX SODAS: 60 teaspoons of sugar and 1,080 calories

The World Health Organization recommends that no more than 10 percent of your daily calories come from sugar. So if you consume 2,000 calories a day, no more than 200 of your calories should come from sugar, and it takes about 50 grams, or roughly 12½ teaspoons, of sugar to amount to 200 calories. Be mindful of the amount of sugar you add to your food, but also check the list of ingredients on grocery store items because sugar can be found in less obvious items like spaghetti sauce. With sugar hidden in so many foods, if you're not careful you can reach 50 grams before you know it. And that amount may even be too much if you're restricting your total calories in an effort to lose weight (see Item #15).

Cutting down on packaged, processed, and prepared foods will help you reduce the amount of sugar you consume. Packaged food often contains hidden sugars in the form of glucose or fructose, or sugar alcohols such as maltitol, sorbitol, and erythritol. To keep it simple, avoid products that have ingredients ending in *ose* and *ol*, or even better, steer clear of overly processed foods altogether. It's easy once you get in the habit.

Unless you're a diabetic or your doctor has specified otherwise, those of you who think you're satisfying your thirst or sweet tooth with artificial sweeteners and prefer diet soda: you may be doing the most harm of all to your body *and* your weight-reducing efforts. I don't expect the biggie food manufacturers to agree with me, but according to the *Journal of*

Commonsense Eating, artificial sugar substitutes are considered a really dumb idea. Take Splenda (or sucralose), for example. Only a small percentage can be absorbed by your body because it doesn't get recognized as food. That's why it has zero calories. Would you eat a cotton ball? Then why on Earth are you eating something that your body doesn't recognize as food? Very few studies have been conducted on the possible side effects of Splenda. A controversial Duke University study published in the *Journal of Toxicology and Environmental Health* reports that Splenda "contributes to obesity, destroys 'good' intestinal bacteria, and prevents prescription drugs from being absorbed." The study was funded by the Sugar Association, so the Splenda folks are disputing the validity of the report. Duke University researchers say the Sugar Association had no input in the study. A well-known grassroots advocacy group called Citizens for Health is using the study findings to try to reverse the FDA approval of Splenda. Who knows how long that will take?

In the meantime, ask yourself why you're using Splenda and other artificial sugar substitutes. Is it because you have a sweet tooth and you think you're satisfying it? You aren't. You're putting your body through a binge-crash cycle and creating a larger problem, a larger ass, and an unhealthier you. But, you may ask, you're drinking diet soda — how can diet soda cause weight gain? According to an eight-year study conducted by the University of Texas, for diet soda drinkers consuming only one or two cans each day, the risk of becoming overweight or obese was 54.5 percent. For regular soda drinkers consuming that same amount, the risk of being overweight or obese was considerably lower, at 32.8 percent. Those are both dismal odds, but you diet soda drinkers actually have a higher chance of getting fat. Why? Because you can't fool your body. Experts suggest that diet drinks may actually stimulate your appetite. As reported on CBS.com, Leslie Bonci, MPH, RD, of the University of Pittsburgh Medical Center, states the following: "Our bodies are smarter than we think. People think they can just fool the body. But maybe the body isn't fooled. If you are not giving your body those calories you promised it, maybe your body will retaliate by wanting more calories."

Splenda may also be responsible for your moodiness, anxiety, and signs of depression. I have to say "may" because I'm not a Harvard lab rat. However, my teenage daughter went through a Splenda period and was so cranky that only a mother could have loved her, but I can't say that I liked her very much. If you're hooked on Splenda and experiencing any unusual symptoms, like those I just mentioned or others such as bloating, gas, diarrhea, or nausea, try a little test. Give it up for two straight weeks and watch a miracle happen. I saw this firsthand when I threw away my daughter's Costco-size box of Splenda. After a couple of weeks of door slamming and the silent treatment, I witnessed something wondrous emanating from my firstborn — a smile! I felt confident that I'd gotten to the core of the problem, decided that I could continue living with her, and threw away her boarding school application. In case you're wondering why I let her have Splenda in the first place, I can explain. First of all, she was seventeen at the time and I'd pretty much lost control of the situation. Second, I allow my kids to go through phases of objectionable behaviors because I know my silence is the absolute fastest way for them to run the course. My daughter's Splenda weeks weren't nearly as insufferable as my son dressing like the Blue Power Ranger for ten weeks straight when he was in kindergarten and karate chopping my leg every chance he got. My legs were as black and blue as his costume.

Speaking of blue things, what about those other packets, the blue ones and pink ones? Bad news too. Haven't enough studies told us they might very well cause cancer? I know: the scientific evidence is inconclusive and everything causes cancer and you're going to die eventually anyway. That argument drives me nuts! Why do you wear your seatbelt, then? Because you are decreasing the chances of dying in a car accident. So decrease your chances of dying because of the rotten choices you're making. I know what some of you are thinking: you only wear your seatbelt (or your bike or motorcycle helmet) because it's the law. The reason stupid laws like that exist is that some of us can't make good decisions for ourselves, so someone has to make them for us. It's time to become a better decision maker.

The next time you have the urge for a regular soda, a diet soda, an energy drink, or a sports drink, drink a glass of water instead. When we are thirsty or dehydrated, our body needs water. How much do we need? Medical opinions vary, but the consensus appears to be somewhere around eight cups a day, or half your weight in ounces — meaning a 150-pound person should aim for seventy-five ounces of water per day. Keep in mind that most fruits and vegetables contain water as well. I also count tea toward my total daily water intake. Clear urine is an indicator that you're getting enough water.

Not only does water keep you hydrated; it helps your digestive system function properly and enables you to maintain optimum metabolism. Water consumption also helps to keep your skin hydrated and moist, which is becoming more and more important to me now that I'm over forty. When you drink soda in place of water, you are robbing your body of something it desperately needs. Reversing just this one habit will make a big difference in your quest to lose the fat and become a healthier you. To make your dining-out experiences more festive and to help wean you from the soda habit, ask your server to add a lemon, lime, cucumber, or orange wedge to your water glass for added flavor.

Whether you're dining out or at home, be sure to drink purified, filtered water so you're not unknowingly taking small doses of someone else's Viagra or Prozac. A staggering number of pharmaceuticals are regularly found in public drinking water. Although a bit spendy, installing a home water purification and filtration system is an excellent idea. Those plastic water bottles that are sold just about everywhere don't necessarily contain purified, filtered water. They might actually be less healthy for you than regular tap water because water bottle companies aren't required to test for pathogens, and worse, they are creating a giant waste problem. Eric Yaverbaum, cofounder of Tappening.com, says every year, America uses 17 million barrels of crude oil to produce plastic bottles, and 38 billion bottles end up in landfills. Tappening's recent ad campaign slogan is "Get off the bottle. Advocate tap." Carry a thermos or stainless steel or aluminum water bottle when you're out and about. If you forget and find yourself in a dehydration pinch, be sure to recycle plastic bottles to cut down on landfill volume and decrease the amount of resources required to make more new plastic crap.

Okay, I think you've got the message to drink water and not diet soda or regular soda, but what about that nagging sweet tooth? Your craving for sweets is your body looking for energy. So give it energy — fuel it up! See Item #12 for a bunch of suggestions for healthy snacks. I have trained myself to consume only what my body can use to maintain a healthy me. I have made this a habit, one that I follow easily and effortlessly, and so can you. Soda pop, artificial sweeteners, and any foods containing high fructose corn syrup are not on the List.

I'm sorry to say, that includes chewing gum. Most popular brands of sugary chewing gum contain high fructose corn syrup. Sugar-free chewing gum is full of potentially harmful sugar substitutes like Splenda (sucralose), Equal (aspartame), NutraSweet (aspartame), or Sweet'N Low (saccharin). I haven't found one that doesn't stick to my overabundance of dental work, but there are natural chewing gum options; just be sure to read the labels carefully.

Try your favorite foods unsweetened. Did you know that a perfectly ripened grapefruit tastes amazing all by itself? Introduce yourself to what food really tastes like. You'll be surprised. The more you do this, the less dependent you'll be on sweeteners and the better you'll feel. If you need to add sweetener to something, such as a cup of coffee or tea, a bowl of cereal, or a cup of plain yogurt, use a small amount of raw brown sugar, raw honey, real maple syrup, or my personal favorite, agave nectar.

Agave nectar is a terrific sweetener. Just ask Jose Cuervo — he's a big fan of the blue agave plant, which is the source of the nectar. I use it to sweeten my tea or coffee and often in recipes that call for sugar. It's about one and a half times sweeter than refined sugar, and it's less viscous than honey so is not nearly as messy to deal with.

The best part about agave nectar is it metabolizes slowly and doesn't spike your blood sugar (insulin level). We've all heard, "it's calories in, calories out," right? It's true that a deficit will cause weight loss, while a surplus will cause weight gain. If I severely restricted my daily calorie intake, but my diet consisted solely of refined cane sugar, I seriously doubt I'd lose weight because I'd be sending my blood sugar (insulin level) through the roof. According to Barbara Berkeley, MD, a board-certified internist who has specialized in treating overweight and obese patients for over twenty years, "insulin is the hormone that opens your fat cells and allows foods to be stored as fat. It is the only major hormone that has this job." So you want to keep your insulin level low *and* keep calories in check to accumulate less fat. (More on this in Item #2.) Even though maple syrup also metabolizes slowly, I reach for the agave nectar more often because the flavor is less strong and I can use it with a variety of foods.

Another alternative to sugar is stevia, an intensely sweet

herb that isn't regulated by the FDA and as of this writing is approved only as a diet supplement. To me, that means the sugar and sugar-substitute manufacturers (like the company that makes Splenda) are likely lobbying the FDA hard to prevent stevia from becoming mainstream and popular and cutting into their share of the business. Stevia comes in a liquid or powder form and can be found at many grocery stores next to the other sweeteners. It's been around for a long time and has zero calories. It has a subtle licorice flavor, so it might take a little getting used to. Stevia comes from the rainforests of Paraguay, is far sweeter than sugar, and doesn't affect your blood sugar levels. The Mayo Clinic website says it may also assist in the treatment of type 2 diabetes and high blood pressure but recommends checking with your doctor before using it.

Barley malt syrup and brown rice syrup are two other whole-food, natural sweeteners that metabolize slowly. I haven't tried these, but only because I'm all about keeping it simple, and agave nectar or going sans sweetener does the trick for me.

Change your mind about sugar and sweets. Retrain yourself, and develop new habits that easily and effortlessly say no to sweets and anything containing HFCS. Tell yourself you don't eat them, and don't. Just as someone who has an allergy to peanuts says, "I don't eat peanuts. They make me really sick," say, "I don't eat gummy bears. They make me really fat." Change your mind, and your habits will follow.

Try this simple experiment. Buy or make your favorite dessert. Put a generous serving on a plate. At home after dinner, have a seat at the dining room table by yourself. Take a bite of your dessert. One bite. Think about how great it tastes — pretty incredible, right? Before you take another bite, think about why you want another bite. You already know what it tastes like. Do you ever really taste anything after the first bite anyway? You've already eaten dinner, so you're not hungry. You've had twenty to thirty seconds of dessert ecstasy. Do you really need another twenty to thirty seconds, or maybe three or four minutes if you decide to eat the entire dessert? We're talking seconds and minutes here. What if you ate just that one bite, savored it, and enjoyed it immensely, and then left it at that? You haven't compromised anything. You won't be any fatter tomorrow than you are today, and you still got to taste that delicious mouthful of dessert. If you eat more of your dessert, it'll just be more of that same taste, but it might not be more of the same in terms of your body — it will likely cause you to get increasingly fatter.

Need a more graphic representation? That one bite has left your mouth and your taste buds. Now what happens? It's on its way to mixing with stomach acids and being broken down and will soon be moving through your gastrointestinal tract, where it will eventually end up as waste. Your body will take all the nutrients it can get from that bite and send them to where they will best serve you. In the case of most desserts, very little can be used to serve, or fuel, your body, so it ends up as doughy filling for your fat cells. One bite, no problem, but the entire dessert can affect your weight.

ITEM #1: YOUR SWEET TOOTH

While you are changing your habits and beginning to retrain yourself, you may every so often want just one bite of something so as not to feel deprived or cheated. Have one bite. And remember what eating more than that can do to your body. It can make you fat. I will be showing you how to make lifelong habits that can easily and effortlessly allow you to reach and maintain your ideal, healthy weight. Some of these changes may be tougher to make than others, so when you are faced with a particularly stubborn bad habit, try the one-bite method. Eventually you'll decide that fattening desserts aren't worth the trouble, and you'll skip them entirely.

ITEM #1: SODA POP, GUMMY BEARS, AND YOUR SWEET TOOTH

1. Avoid any product containing high fructose corn syrup.
2. Pass on regular soda, diet soda, sports drinks, and energy drinks.
3. Use raw, brown sugar or honey as your sweetener, or give sugar alternatives like stevia and agave nectar a try. Avoid artificial sweeteners like Splenda, aspartame, and saccharin. Limit your daily intake of sugar to 10 percent or less of your total calories.
4. Stay hydrated by drinking purified, filtered water (at least half your body weight in ounces daily).
5. Eat just one bite of dessert or skip it altogether.

THE SUMMER
OF MY DISCONTENT

I WAS FEELING PRETTY LOW when I came home from college the summer after my freshman year. I've shared that I was fat and the guy I'd been seeing broke up with me, but that's not all I was sulking about. My academic efforts resulted in a 2.25 cumulative GPA, my Grandma died that spring, and my parents moved while I was away and no longer had a bedroom for me. To make it perfectly clear I was unwelcome in *their* new home (feeling sorry for myself here), during the move, my dad threw out all my personal belongings, including concert T-shirts, gymnastics ribbons, and mementos from high school. I was fat and homeless for the first time in my life. To make matters worse, I cut all my hair off and got a tight perm on what was left. This created a hideous red afro on top of my circle-shaped face, which would have been perfectly round if it hadn't been for the double chin that was starting to form. I was Molly Ringwald's ugly twin sister — the one without a bedroom or personal belongings.

I was also heartbroken and determined to shed the weight, grow my hair out, and get the guy back. Not so quick, my little butterball. That's literally how my dad referred to me that summer. Dear Ol' Dad said I couldn't go back to college in the fall because my grades were so bad. I pleaded with him to give me another chance, and he said the only way I could return in the fall was if I earned enough over the summer to pay for my tuition. He would pick up the rest. It was a deal. I'd always had jobs throughout high school, mostly at retail clothing stores, where I spent my entire paycheck buying clothes with my employee discount. He said that wouldn't work this time around. He was getting me a job. Since they had given my car to my younger brother, I snottily asked how he proposed I would get to this wonderful new opportunity. He had it all figured out: my great aunt Jean was lending me her car for the summer, since her driver's license had been revoked.

Her car was an early-seventies baby blue Mercury Comet with cigarette burn marks all over the vinyl seats. It smelled horrible. The steering wheel was enormous, and the car floated so badly, I had trouble keeping it in one lane on the freeway. I kept to the slow lane and didn't dare take it over 45. It was such an embarrassment that I refused to park it where other people could see me get out. At work that summer, I parked about a half mile away, and everyone just thought I took the bus or someone dropped me off. It's not like I didn't desperately need the exercise.

I rented a room at my best friend's childhood home. Karrie had it made. She had the entire basement to herself — her own family room and TV, a private bathroom, a wet bar, and, thankfully, an extra bedroom. I always got along well with her parents, so I thought it would work out relatively well. Karrie was really excited to have me there. I told her not to get too jacked up. I was on a mission to get back to my thin self, and I informed her that I would not be drinking beer and partying into the wee hours, smoking clove cigarettes, or eating our favorite dish — a massive pile of nachos that consisted of Doritos, ground beef, refried beans, black olives, guacamole, sour cream, and at least three cups of shredded cheddar cheese — which was so huge, we had to put it in a rectangular cake pan. Instead, I would be going to my job, dragging my fat ass to the gym, and eating next to nothing. She hated having me there. Her mom, Caryl, loved it. She'd been trying to lose weight for years and now had someone to walk with, plan meals with, and talk to about weight-loss progress. We became the greatest of buddies.

In fact, Caryl became my only buddy. I was pissed at my parents, Karrie was disgusted at the sight of me, and my self-loathing had turned me into a quiet, introverted, mopey recluse. My new job didn't help matters. I was now a telemarketer for a hardwood company that was located roughly twenty miles from Karrie's house in an industrial area of Portland that I had never known existed. I was to develop a survey to determine what local cabinetmakers and woodworkers thought of the hardwoods we sold to them. I had to start each call with, "Hi, my name is Kami. I'm a freshman communications major at Arizona State University, and I'm calling on behalf of so-and-so." (You'll see in a minute why I can't divulge the name of the business.) I was to ask these customers a series of questions that I had created myself, and at the end of the summer, make charts and graphs summarizing the data. Easy enough, right? Wrong. Cabinetmakers and woodworkers are a bunch of cranks. They were appallingly mean to me on the phone. After a few calls, I couldn't take it anymore. I already felt like crap about myself, and I wasn't about to let a bunch of grouchy old men make me feel any worse. I couldn't quit, so I did the only thing I could think of: I faked it. I spent the next twelve weeks pretending to be on the phone. And in the end, I made some beautiful and colorful charts and graphs showing how happy the customers were with their hardwood products.

Since I "worked" alone and was otherwise antisocial, I hadn't gotten to know the two staff secretaries. They were both really pretty and skinny, so I decided I wouldn't like them anyway. On my last day, they asked if they could take me to lunch. My hair had grown out a little, and I had lost a considerable amount of weight, thanks to daily aerobics and Caryl's brown-bag lunches and dinner salads, so I was feeling a bit more jovial by this point. We went to Old Town Pizza, where they ordered pepperoni pizza and pitchers of beer and got me drunk. Then they asked me how my job had gone that summer. "Fine. Why?" Oh, because they knew I had faked every call because I had never hit the button that lit up to indicate when one of the phone lines was in use. They thought it was hilarious and cackled hysterically every time I hung up the phone after one of my "calls." I had thought I heard sounds of laughter! The three of us had so much fun that day, and it made me wish I'd befriended them sooner.

But Caryl was my only friend that summer. I thought I was fat and ugly and not deserving of friends or social activities. I realize now how silly that was. A bit psychotic, actually. Here's where I make my point: If you have some weight (or even considerable weight) to lose and are feeling anything remotely like I once did and you're waiting to live your life until after you achieve your weight-loss goals, *stop*. This *is* your life, and as far as we know, you only get one. Get out there and share your triumphs and difficulties with anyone and everyone. People want to know you. Those two secretaries would have liked me fat or thin. We would have had fun together all summer. I could have been laughing with them! Maybe there's a Caryl figure in your life who is just dying to have someone to commiserate with, walk with, eat with, have tea with, and get to know. Likely, there are many "Caryls" and many co-workers, friends, family members, and acquaintances who would love to share some good times with you.

I hope you didn't think that the moral of my story was about being honest in your job — that faking is a form of deceit and you should come clean and make it right. I do have some residual guilt, but I was only trying to encourage you to make some friends, have some fun, and join in on the action, no matter where you are in your weight-loss efforts.

THE GREAT DEBATE

White vs. Brown Carbohydrates, the Glycemic Index, and the Miracle of Fiber

Health is not a matter of chance. It is a matter of choice.
It is something we have been gifted with,
took for granted and we can reclaim and regain.
— Author unknown

ET'S RESOLVE THE GREAT CARBOHYDRATE DEBATE. I have one goal in mind with this chapter: to convince you that eating the right carbohydrates is the secret to losing and maintaining weight and the key to long-term health.

Since carbohydrates have been a significant part of my success in maintaining my weight, I find all this low-carb business particularly fascinating. This is not to suggest that you should eat carbs willy-nilly and they should make up the bulk of your diet. Instead, you should learn to eat only the right carbs, and they should become an integral part of your balanced diet. The Harvard School of Public Health has a terrific nutrition section on its website. In surprisingly plain English, it explains the real deal with carbohydrates and how fad diets such as Atkins, South

Beach, and other low-carb plans have "led many Americans to believe that carbohydrates are bad, the source of unflattering flab and a cause of the obesity epidemic." They go on (and on and on) to say how that type of thinking is a "dangerous oversimplification." Robert H. Eckel, MD, director of the general clinical research center at the University of Colorado Health Sciences Center, tells WebMD.com, "Our worries over the Atkins Diet go way past the question of whether it is effective for losing weight or even for keeping weight off. We worry that the diet promotes heart disease. We have concerns over whether this is a healthy diet for preventing heart disease, stroke, and cancer. There is also potential loss of bone, and the potential for people with liver and kidney problems to have trouble with the high amounts of protein in these diets."

This chapter is a biggie. Suck it up, because this whole carb thing is vitally important to your success in weight loss and weight maintenance. I've bookended this chapter with personal stories on purpose so you'll be at least mildly entertained before and after reading about why you should rethink carbs starting right now. So let's get to it.

Not all carbohydrates are equal. I repeat, not all carbohydrates are equal. This may be the understatement of the year or even the decade. I'm not saying more than a decade because one of you will undoubtedly think of a worse understatement, like "butter sure has a lot of fat in it." One cup of butter has 1,628 calories. Guess how many of those calories come from fat? 1,628! I'm no mathematician, but that seems like all of them. I go off about this because my friend's boyfriend (at the time) once asked me at dinner if butter really has that much fat in it. I was so dumbfounded, I couldn't answer and just snarled up my face. Later, in private, I asked my girlfriend whether this relationship could really go anywhere.

But back to the carbs. While refined, simple, and starchy carbohydrates, such as white bread, white rice, white potatoes, white pasta, and highly processed foods, can contribute to weight gain and can prevent weight loss, whole grains (aka complex carbohydrates) found in foods like whole wheat bread, whole wheat pasta, and brown rice can have the opposite effect. Not only are they the key to weight loss and weight maintenance; they can also reduce your risk of heart disease and diabetes. Not to be overlooked are legumes (beans), fruits, and vegetables, which are also carbohydrate superstars.

White bread, white pasta, white rice, and white potatoes are an extremely inefficient source of fuel for your body. These "white" foods raise your body's sugar levels instantly, but only for a brief period of time. Whole grains, on the other hand, raise your body's sugar levels gradually and sustain them over a long period of time. Basically, you feel full for a lot longer. If you're thinking that's not important, think again. Feeling full and satisfied prevents us from overeating or eating the wrong foods, which in turn can prevent us from getting fat.

Have you heard of the glycemic index? Instead of classifying carbohydrates as merely simple or complex, the glycemic index scores carbs on a scale of 0 to 100 based on how quickly and how high they boost blood sugar (insulin levels) as compared with pure glucose, which has a score of 100. This will be easiest for golfers to comprehend, since the low scores are the best scores. Carbohydrates with a glycemic-index (GI) score of 70 or higher are considered high-GI, while those scoring less than 55 are considered low-GI. The ones in the middle are, you guessed it, medium-GI carbohydrates. To put that in perspective, your average baked potato has a GI score of 85, whereas brown rice has a score of 55. Only carbohydrates can have a GI score; foods consisting solely of protein or fat will not have one. This GI business matters to your weight-loss success because of what I mentioned in the first chapter: insulin allows your body to create fat storage, so you want to keep your insulin levels low to accumulate less fat. Interestingly, fat and protein don't stimulate your body to make a significant amount of insulin.

Whole grains have low GI scores. They are digested slowly and don't spike your insulin levels. White, processed foods and grains, white potatoes, and sugar have high GI scores and have the opposite effect. Here's another example. White sandwich bread has a GI score of 71 (high), whereas its brown, whole grain counterpart has a GI score of 51 (low). The white bread will cause a greater and faster spike to your insulin or sugar levels than the whole grain variety. Again, insulin allows your body to create fat storage, so ditch the white, processed foods, candy, soda pop, ice cream, and hundreds of other high-GI foods, and keep your insulin levels low if you want to give the calories you consume the greatest chance of burning off and not being stored as fat — the kind of fat that likes to congregate around your belly, your ass, and your thighs. See why white, starchy, processed foods are not on the List?

The glycemic load (GL) further complicates things by providing another score based on how *much* of the carbohydrate you consume. For example, eating one small piece of high-GI candy won't do much to your blood sugar levels because it's such a meager amount that your body won't respond too significantly. That piece of candy may have a high GI score but at the same time have a low GL score based on the serving size. To keep things simple, I pretty much ignore the whole glycemic load business and only consume carbohydrates that have low GI scores so I don't have to worry about it. If you stick to whole grains, you won't have to pay much attention to specific GI scores, either, but in case you're interested, the University of Sydney in Australia has created a handy database of the GI scores of over sixteen hundred carbohydrates, at Glycemicindex.com.

In addition to interfering with weight loss and putting you at an increased risk for diabetes and heart disease, white, starchy, high-GI carbohydrates are low in fiber. Fiber is your friend — a consistent friend you can count on when you need one. If you're not getting my delicate innuendo, fiber keeps you regular! Fiber is indigestible complex carbohydrates. Our body can't break fiber down. Instead of being used for energy, fiber goes through our intestines and acts like a broom, sweeping and cleaning along its way to becoming waste.

There are two kinds of fiber: soluble and insoluble. This is where it gets a bit gross, but insoluble fiber doesn't dissolve in water and remains largely unchanged as it passes through your digestive tract. I think we all know at least one food that contains insoluble fiber — bright yellow corn, right? I'm sure all you diaper changers can think of a few more. Insoluble fiber scours the walls of your intestines and removes waste matter. The other kind, soluble fiber, dissolves in water, lowers bad cholesterol, and slows down the digestive process (specifically, the absorption of glucose). Slow digestion is your new best friend. Many foods contain soluble and insoluble fiber, and both types are critical for good health and weight loss and maintenance. In addition to having low GI scores, whole grains are typically high in fiber.

The good news is, every white, starchy, high-GI food has a brown, low-GI counterpart. The key to these brown carbohydrates isn't actually their color. It's that they are "whole," meaning they have not been processed to remove all the nutrients. In 2006, the FDA finally got around to defining the term *whole grain*: "whole grain foods should contain the three key ingredients of cereal grains — bran (the fiber-filled outer part of the kernel), endosperm (the inner part and usually all that is left in most processed grains), and the germ (the heart of the grain kernel.)" In an effort to quash any creative interpretations, the FDA stipulates not only that all three ingredients (the bran, the endosperm, and the germ) need to be present but also that they must be present in the same relative proportion that they naturally exist in, thereby preventing clever food manufacturers from just adding a little bran and germ to highly processed foods.

Do whole grain sandwich bread, brown rice, whole wheat pasta, whole wheat bagels, and whole grain hamburger and hotdog buns sound like a real stretch for you? It just takes a little training — training yourself to see foods differently until it becomes a habit. Habits are easy and require little, if any, effort. Whole grain foods fuel your body. They keep it running. They will help your body become healthy and lean. Your body uses every milligram of them to your benefit. Whole grains will help you lose the fat.

For lunch today, or tomorrow if it's already past lunchtime, have a sandwich on whole grain bread. Pile it high with your favorites — or better yet, my favorites: turkey, avocado, lettuce, tomato, and Dijon mustard. Have a whole sandwich — a nice big sandwich. If you want a little mayo, use it sparingly, or try one of the lower-fat mayonnaises or one made using canola oil instead of eggs. Skip the cheese. Don't eat meat? No sweat. There is nothing more satisfying that a peanut butter and jelly sandwich. Almond butter is tasty too. But make sure your peanut or almond butter contains only one ingredient: ground peanuts or almonds. In fact, all the items you buy at the grocery store should have very few ingredients. The fewer, the better for you. Your jelly should be a 100 percent real-fruit spread. I make my own single-ingredient jam by mashing up fresh or frozen strawberries, blueberries, raspberries, or blackberries. Another non-meat option is a vegetable sandwich layered with hummus.

Don't knock it 'til you try it. (If you have a dining companion, just make sure they eat the same thing because hummus has some serious garlic in it!)

Need something to go on the side? No problem, but chips are not on the List. You get something better — better for your waistline and better for your body — *soup*! A cup of tomato-based, broth-based, or legume-based soup is the perfect complement to your sandwich. Tomato is my personal favorite. Not a soup person? Well, you should change your mind about soup. Soup is your friend. However, there *are* "bad" soups, or soups that should be eaten in very small doses: cream-based soups. New England clam chowder and lobster bisque are not on the List. I'm lazy and go for what's readily available, but if you're willing to put in a little effort, there are plenty of recipes for lower-fat versions of chowders and bisques.

You could also have a bowl of fresh fruit or a tossed salad with your sandwich. For tossed salads, skip the croutons. If you must use cheese, use only a tiny amount, like real Parmesan (which does not come in a can, folks), and toss your salad with a small amount of dressing before putting it on your plate. This ensures that every bite tastes good and prevents you from adding more dressing.

Let's talk about your salad dressing for a moment. You will do your body a world of good if you train yourself to get excited about the taste of the salad ingredients rather than the dressing you're going to drown them in. Buy yourself a nice bottle of balsamic vinegar. Whisk it together with olive oil, fresh or dried herbs, freshly ground pepper, and a touch of sea salt, and then ever so lightly dress your salad. Then toss the crap out of it. If you're completely hung up on cream-based dressings like blue cheese or ranch, you get to use even less dressing. A lot less. But salads don't require a ton of dressing. Make it your mission to taste all the delicious ingredients in your salad, and don't smother them in dressing — no more than one tablespoon, and give it a good toss.

Be creative with your salad. Include a variety of items: green onions (scallions), carrots, celery, beets, garbanzo beans (chickpeas), corn, hard-boiled eggs, a few chopped almonds or walnuts, avocado, black beans, salsa, black olives, mandarin oranges, apples, radishes, mushrooms, tomatoes, grapes, dried cranberries, and the like. Try a variety of leafy greens, including spinach, arugula, kale, Swiss chard, and red leaf, butter, baby, and romaine lettuce. Dark green, leafy vegetables like spinach help you get your daily dose of vitamin K, which helps reduce inflammation. According to RealAge.com, inflammation is "super bad" for your body and is thought to be a contributor to heart problems like cardiovascular disease and heart attacks.

Go easy on healthy but high-calorie items like raw nuts, avocados, and olives. Monster salads, available at many chain restaurants, seem like the ideal choice, but watch out for an endless supply of less-healthy, higher-fat items like candied nuts and bacon bits. Those seemingly light meals can easily add up to the fat-and-calorie equivalent of a Big Mac.

Wash your lunch down with a delicious, tall glass of water. By the end of your lunch, make sure you've finished the entire glass. In time, eating every sandwich with whole grain bread will become a habit, a delicious habit that you will follow easily and effortlessly.

Let's not stop there. Make every piece of toast, every pancake, every pita pocket, every cracker, every noodle, every English muffin, every tortilla, every bowl of cereal, every dinner roll — you get the point — whole grain or whole wheat. And that's not just wheat, but *whole* wheat. When the list of ingredients says *wheat* or *enriched wheat*, this is just a watered-down version of whole wheat and is virtually no better for you than the starchy, white kind. *Enriched* means that important vitamins and minerals were lost in the processing and were added back in to make your food healthier. They shouldn't have been removed in the first place! You don't want your grains processed; you want them left intact and whole.

Other good options for whole grains include oat, barley, rye, linseed, millet, brown rice, spelt, quinoa (more on this one in a minute), and kamut. If you see the words *multigrain* or *cracked wheat* on a product label, check the list of ingredients and make sure the word *whole* appears before the name of any grains listed. You may want to try sprouted grain breads, especially if you're intolerant of gluten (or wheat). I know *sprouted grain* sounds a little odd — like when you were five and your dad told you that you'd grow a watermelon in your stomach if you swallowed the seeds (please tell me I'm not the only one whose dad said that). Not to worry — the sprouting occurs *before* the grain enters your body. When grains are sprouted, your body can more easily absorb the important vitamins like folic acid, thiamine, and good old vitamin C. *Stone ground* is another term you may encounter. This is a method of grinding whole grains between two slowly moving stones. It requires less heat and preserves valuable nutrients, which are typically lost in conventional, high-speed milling. Did you know that getting two or more servings of whole grains every day could reduce your risk of pancreatic cancer by as much as forty percent? That's what researchers at the University of California discovered. They also found that eating two or more doughnuts each week puts you at an increased risk for this type of cancer. As a general rule, get in the habit of reading the labels on packaged foods. When shopping for grain-based foods, look at the list of ingredients and make sure the first item listed is a whole grain and that you recognize every item.

Okay, this next one may be tougher for you than switching from white bread to whole grain bread: white potatoes are not on the List. (My Swedish grandpa would disown me for saying so if he were still alive. I doubt the potatoes were responsible for his death ... but then again, Grandpa thoroughly enjoyed his nightly vodka tonics. If I'm not mistaken, vodka is often made from potatoes, and Gramps died of cirrhosis of the liver, so perhaps it *was* Death by Potato!) Potatoes have a high GI score, spike your sugar levels instantly, and don't sustain you or fill you up. I eat sweet potatoes and yams, which have a low GI score, and pile 'em high with healthy toppings like green onions, black beans, and a touch of lowfat sour cream. Baked sweet potato "fries" are a delicious substitute for French fries. (See Item #9, page 126, for a quick and simple recipe.)

Pasta is an easy one. There are many varieties of whole wheat pasta at your grocery store. To get used to it, start out with basic whole wheat spaghetti with a tomato-based sauce. Add Italian chicken sausage if you eat meat and want something more substantial. The coloring in the sauce hides the noodles' brownish hue, and the sauce is zesty and flavorful to help you ease into the difference in texture and flavor. I don't think it's that different, but some of you might. My kids are major whiners, and when they were younger, they had no idea that they were eating whole wheat pasta at our house and white pasta at their friends' homes. Try whole wheat lasagna next. I pile mine high with chicken basil sausage, pesto sauce, chopped walnuts, a light amount of Parmesan and Gorgonzola cheese, and sautéed garlic, onions, mushrooms, and spinach — always a crowd pleaser. Other whole grain pasta options are spelt, brown rice, and corn varieties. If that sounds too health food store–freakish to you, those are just grains in the form of tasty noodles that you can find at your average grocery store. When you cook them just right and toss them with a Bolognese or marinara sauce and freshly grated Parmesan cheese, you'll be in pasta paradise. Soba noodles, often found in Japanese dishes, are made from buckwheat and are reasonably high in protein and low on the glycemic index but less than impressive in the fiber department. When it comes to pasta sauce, opt for red over white. Red sauces are typically tomato-based, whereas white sauces are cream-based and are higher in calories and fat.

Replacing white rice with brown rice is a snap. Brown rice, wild rice, or brown basmati rice makes for a great pilaf and tastes terrific with Thai or Indian food. Wheat berries, barley, whole wheat couscous, chia, and quinoa are other good alternatives to white rice. Chia has been given an absurd rap thanks to the Chia pet, "As Seen on TV." Fiber-rich chia seeds date back thousands of years and were a staple food of the Aztecs and the Mayans. They also contain a significant amount of omega-3 fatty acids and antioxidants, which we'll get into a bit later on.

My favorite whole grain is quinoa. Quinoa has a low GI score and is high in fiber and protein. The word is pronounced "KEEN-wa," which sounds exotic and will impress your friends at dinner parties. Just say it's a Peruvian grain that you like to throw in a dish here and there — the high-fiber, low-GI part can be mentioned when you get together with your buddies for coffee. It tastes nutty and delicious. I put it in soup, throw it on salads, make pilaf out of it, and add it to my enchiladas.

So wipe those starchy, white foods out of your mind forever. Poof. Gone. Along with your fat. Tell yourself you don't eat white, starchy foods, and don't. Period. If you closed this book right now and never picked it up again and only followed what I've presented so far — taking just one bite of your dessert or skipping it entirely; avoiding products like soda pop and other sweets that contain refined sugar or high fructose corn syrup;

avoiding artificial sweeteners; and eating whole grain, low-GI foods instead of their white, starchy, high-GI counterparts — you would be well on your way to losing weight, having more energy, and being considerably healthier. But stay with me — there are many more good habits to develop, and I have faith in you. You can retrain yourself. You can change the way you look at food. You can develop new, healthy habits, which will easily and effortlessly help you to lose the fat, forever.

Case in point: Less than a year ago, a good friend of mine, whom I dine with a lot, drank three or four Cokes a day, ate white bread, ate hash browns with his eggs on the weekends, and ate ice cream and gummy bears while he watched his favorite shows. He also didn't eat breakfast during the week. Every so often, he would complain that he was getting a little soft in the belly. Other times he would complain about being tired and low on energy. I asked him if this extra padding on his midsection and this lack of energy could maybe, just possibly, be related to his eating habits. He said he didn't think so. When I offered some suggestions, he said whole wheat bread was too dry and water didn't quench his thirst like Coke did and that he didn't have time to eat a proper breakfast in the morning. I responded with, "Maybe you just need some toughen-up pills." I did say that, but just to make him laugh — which it did not.

I was patient with him and subtly challenged him to make some "slight" changes. It took a few months, but he now eats only whole grain breads and skips the hash browns with his weekend breakfast. And — drum roll, please — he quit drinking Coke. He first reduced his soda intake to one a day and now passes on the dreadful stuff altogether. He also eats breakfast every morning with foods that are on the List (see Item #7). He still has gummy bears and ice cream occasionally, but he's made some major improvements in his eating habits, which is good news for me — I haven't had to listen to his bellyaching since.

ITEM #2: THE GREAT DEBATE

1.   Eat only "brown," low-glycemic, whole grain breads — for sandwiches, hamburger buns, dinner rolls, baguettes, pancakes, waffles, French toast, crackers, et cetera. Read labels carefully and watch out for "enriched" wheat and packaged foods that don't list a whole grain as the first ingredient.
2.   Eat plenty of high-fiber foods every day.
3.   Eat broth-based, tomato-based, and legume-based soups.
4.   Be creative with your salads, go easy on the dressing and cheese, and skip the croutons and candied nuts. Watch out for monster salads at chain restaurants.
5.   Try a variety of whole grains, such as quinoa, barley, wheat berries, and whole wheat couscous.
6.   Switch from regular, white potatoes to sweet potatoes or yams.
7.   Switch from white pasta to whole wheat pasta.
8.   Switch from white rice to brown rice, wild rice, or brown basmati rice.

WHAT MOTIVATES YOU?

MY OLDER SISTER WAS A CHUBBY KID, and except during a few brief periods of dieting, she was always overweight as an adult. For years, she attributed this to not caring about her appearance and being unwilling to deprive herself of certain foods just to look good. Being the unsympathetic younger sister that I can admittedly be at times, I thought it sounded like excuse making, which runs mighty deep in our family. Trying to be helpful, I kindly pointed out that maybe if she got off the couch and made better food choices, she wouldn't have to make righteous declarations about not caring about her appearance.

I recognize now that it's not that simple for some people, like my sister. She now admits that she was eating food for the wrong reasons. Her real motivation was instant gratification, emotional pacification, and boredom. Took her long enough, but finally she understood that she was tired and moody and felt like she was trudging through deep snow all the time because of her diet (her words). As she got older, her back and joints were a regular source of pain and frustration. She felt like crap because she ate like crap.

Early last year, my sister was driving in her car and heard a piece on National Public Radio about a study conducted in London in which the participants went on a Paleo diet. No, this is not a diet for dinosaurs. My sister teaches college science, so this piqued her interest. This Paleo diet supposedly mimicked what early humans would have eaten, which was mostly nuts and seeds, roots, and fruits and vegetables with a bit of fish and meat thrown in once in a while. Something finally clicked for my sister, and I can assure you it wasn't the heels of her adorable shoes because she likely had on ugly brown hiking boots.

This Paleo diet has some similarities to the List, but there are a few major differences: the Paleo diet doesn't include grains, dairy, or legumes. Although participants reported having more energy, better health, and lower weight and feeling more alert and happy, my sister was doubtful that she could maintain such a restrictive diet and be optimally healthy without whole grains, lowfat dairy, or beans and lentils. So she made a few modifications in order to achieve a more balanced diet. It worked. Uh, call me Captain Obvious, but what does she think I've been eating right in front of her for all these years?

After about three months, I noticed she was considerably thinner. At six months, even thinner still. Three months later, she was thin. Thinner than I am! I observed her at family dinners and brunches — no more cubes of cheese and handfuls of crackers or cookies, and no more eating while lounging on the couch. The weight is still off, and I can bet it's gone forever. She finally figured it out. She retrained herself and changed the way she thinks about food. She replaced her old unhealthy, fat-making habits with new healthy, fat-losing habits. She can't believe she waited forty-three years! She's officially thin and has managed to keep the weight off for nearly two years now.

What I enjoy is how our entire family likes to seize every opportunity to remind me that my sister is now thinner than I am. She and I went shopping recently for jeans at Buffalo Exchange (a chain resale shop specializing in current, trendy clothing at killer deals) and we were not competing for the same great finds because she wears a smaller size! I find it interesting that my dear sister always claimed that she didn't care about fashion or looking cute in her jeans because she's not vain like I am. Hmmmm? That's not what I witnessed on our shopping spree. I saw my sister having fun! Busted! I know, the little green monster just entered the room, but I liked being the skinnier and considerably younger sister. Okay, I'm only two years (and two months) younger and I'm really happy for Kelly. Oops, I mentioned her name. (As a side note, want to hear something funny? My sister was born Kelly Gray. She married Mr. Brown, and things went south, literally — he moved to Southern California. Then she married Mr. Ballew, which if you say really quickly sounds like "blue." I bet my brother-in-law would get a little unnerved if Kelly were a bit too flirtatious with a Mr. Green, Mr. White, or Mr. Black. You see what I'm saying?)

Harmless kidding aside, she really is a new person. She used to be quiet and brooding, and now she's outgoing and lights up the room with her smile and cheeriness. It's really annoying. I mean, it's really awesome! Last Christmas, she was literally the life of the party, a role I used to have . . . ahhh, more jealousy and bitterness. Did I mention Kelly was an accident? True story. Wait — I had a point here, and it wasn't that I'm a rotten sister (that one should be fairly obvious by now). My point was that Kelly retrained herself, now sees food as fuel, and has developed habits that easily and effortlessly will keep her body lean and free of excess fat. And I *am* happy for her. Really. So happy that I've included some fantastic recipes in the back of the book that Kelly created. Such an overachiever.

ORGANICALLY SPEAKING

Healthy Organic Food Practices vs. Conventional Food Manufacturing

> *Every human being is the author of his own health or disease.*
> — Buddha

I KNOW ORGANIC FOOD CAN BE MORE EXPENSIVE, and maybe you think it's a giant waste of money. Some of you might even believe eating organic food is akin to being unpatriotic and that the entire organic movement is all propaganda, just like global warming. Sarcasm aside, whatever your issue is with eating organic, let me put in my two cents: eating organic foods won't turn you into a hippie or a liberal activist, and it won't make you suddenly desire a tattoo or a nose ring. The biggest statement it makes about you is that you care deeply about your health and you'd rather not consume poison.

The National Organic Program, run by the United States Department of Agriculture (USDA), regulates and certifies organic foods. "Certified Organic" means that your produce, eggs, meat, and poultry are not raised using antibiotics or growth hormones or produced using pesticides, commercial fertilizers, synthetic ingredients, sewage sludge, bioengineering, or ionizing radiation. In addition, organically raised animals that produce meat and dairy products must be treated humanely and given access to the outdoors and fresh air. For a farm's products to be labeled organic, a government-approved certifier inspects the farm to make sure the products meet USDA organic standards. The USDA even takes it a step further, requiring that "companies that handle or process organic food before it gets to your local supermarket or restaurant must be certified, too." Your body cannot use chemicals, pesticides, hormones, and by-products of sewage sludge to its benefit; they act only to its detriment. Sewage sludge? Sick. I say, stop poisoning yourself and your family, reduce your chances of getting cancer and other ailments, pay the extra money, have more peace of mind, and try to eat organic as often as possible. I provide some cost-cutting strategies later in this chapter.

Certified-organic food is produced on ecologically friendly farms that are required to use sustainable practices that ensure the use of renewable resources and the conservation of soil and water, which keeps your drinking water cleaner. According to the Union of Concerned Scientists, sustainable farming practices mean "treating the farm as an integrated whole composed of soil, plants, animals, and insects whose interaction can be adjusted and enriched to solve problems and maximize yields."

The social movement known as "fair trade" promotes

sustainability while simultaneously striving to ease global poverty by advocating fair prices and better environmental conditions for workers in developing countries that grow food staples such as coffee, cocoa, sugar, tea, and fruit. The fair-trade movement's intent is to improve the economic self-sufficiency of the workers and growers and to give them greater equity in the global market. Look for the "Fair Trade" label along with the "Certified Organic" label.

One tiny word of caution: just because a food is certified organic doesn't mean you should eat it. There are hundreds of organic foods that are not on the List: white hamburger buns, Yukon gold potatoes, and chocolate ice cream will never be yes foods. Also keep in mind that some organic farms are located near conventional farms, and cross contamination can occur. Make sure to wash meat and produce items thoroughly to remove any synthetic residue like pesticides.

Genetically modified organisms (GMOs) are another thing to look out for, only you want to avoid them like the plague instead of seeking them out. GMOs are plant-based foods whose genetic makeup, or DNA, has been altered. That's a simplified explanation, but you get the idea: food scientists are messing with plant life that has been in existence for thousands, or in some cases millions, of years. They do this mainly so plants (including grains) will become resistant to bugs, viruses, weather, or predators. The fact that we're messing with Mother Nature scares me silly. Fortunately, for foods to be certified organic, they cannot contain GMOs. However, in conventionally produced foods (that is, foods that aren't certified organic), GMOs are not regulated or tested, and the producers are not required to label the food as genetically modified. GMOs have been available in plant-based foods in the United States since the mid-nineties and are linked to a variety of health problems, including resistance to antibiotics and an increase in food allergies.

The website of the social and environmental activism organization Care2 suggests that even though there is currently no sure way to avoid GMOs, eating foods that are certified organic is your best bet. However, even that is not an absolute guarantee, as farmers may unknowingly buy genetically engineered seeds because, again, no labeling is required. The brilliant editors of *E/The Environmental Magazine* have a smokin'-hot tip in their book, *Green Living*: Look at the PLU codes of the produce you're buying. PLU codes that begin with the number 8 are genetically modified; those beginning with the number 9 are grown organically; and those beginning with the number 4 have been grown using conventional methods. That helps with produce, but what about cereal, bread, and other items containing grains? For now, the best advice I can give you is buy only certified-organic products, stage a protest, and stay tuned.

The editors of *Green Living* also suggest shopping the perimeter of your grocery store, where all the fresh food is located, like fruits, vegetables, seafood, and meats. The packaged, processed, and frozen foods are typically found in the center of the store. They add that this could also be a money-saving strategy, since fresh foods typically cost less than processed foods. Want another money-saving strategy? Grow your own organic vegetables! If you already love gardening, try your hand at growing organic tomatoes, lettuce, herbs, berries, and all sorts of other tasty plant-based foods. Be daring and try some heirloom varieties. (I say this, but I have to admit I have zero experience cultivating my own food. I don't have to, because I have numerous family members who love to garden and know I'm lazy and deathly afraid of worms and slugs and can't remember to water my plants. They bring me samples of their plentiful bounty on a regular basis.)

Buying in bulk whenever possible is another terrific idea because it cuts down on excessive packaging and saves you money. Many grocery stores sell a variety of organic items in bulk, including cereal, grains, and nuts. For bulk-aisle shopping, either bring your own bags or containers or use brown paper bags from the produce section and reuse them several times before recycling them. Some stores, the ones that don't specialize in organic foods, stock organic items in the health and natural foods aisle. Keep in mind that *natural* and *organic* do not mean the same thing. This may change soon, but for now, *natural* is not a regulated term, whereas *organic* is. Also, be on the lookout for the label "contains organic ingredients." That doesn't mean *all* the ingredients are organic or that the product is certified by the USDA and meets organic standards. Other labels you may encounter are for specific foods like coffee and wine. Here in the Pacific Northwest, wines that are produced with little or no impact on nearby rivers are given a "Salmon Safe" label. For coffee, the Rainforest Alliance certifies thousands of farms, on over a million acres in nineteen countries, that use sustainable farming practices, conserving water and soil and protecting wildlife and the welfare of their workers.

Make sure your food supply travels the shortest distance possible. The more you eat organic food that is locally grown and produced, the less energy and fewer resources are required to feed you. As the June 2008 issue of *Wired* magazine reminds us, not all organic food is grown by Farmer John — much of it comes from agribusiness giants that make organic food and then ship it thousands of miles in "refrigerator trucks belching carbon-dioxide" so you can buy it at your local grocery store. This is one reason that farmers' markets are the best idea since sliced bread (whole wheat, of course). Spending money at farmers' markets tells the farmers to continue to put their land to good use and keep growing healthy food for the local population. Food that comes from a nearby farm is going to taste a lot fresher and better than food that has traveled hundreds or thousands of miles. You can also feel good because you are supporting the local economy.

Patronizing farmers' markets and buying local and seasonal food sends a powerful message not only to small, nearby farmers but also to the entire food-manufacturing industry. You are one person and you have considerable power. Every dime you spend on organic, local, seasonal, fair-trade, non-GMO food grown using sustainable practices communicates to the food industry what kind of product is in demand.

ITEM #3: ORGANICALLY SPEAKING

To locate farmers' markets, food co-ops, restaurants, bakeries, and personal chefs that provide local, sustainable, and organic food, go to Eatwellguide.org and enter your zip code for a complete listing by category. If farmers' markets or nearby fruit stands don't exist where you live, read labels carefully at the grocery store to determine where the organic products you purchase have been produced, and opt for those that have traveled the shortest distance.

Have you heard the term *clean eating?* Because we are so label-obsessed in this country, the concept of eating local and seasonal food that has been minimally processed and doesn't contain artificial ingredients now has a name. For those of you who enjoy labels and like to keep up with the latest trends, eating foods on the List sort of, kind of, almost enrolls you in the Clean Eaters Club (not to be confused with the Clean Your Plate Club, which for obvious reasons I would encourage you to drop out of, effective immediately). Please note that I'm not 100 percent behind the clean eating movement because I checked out *Clean Eating* magazine and its website, and while the recipes and accompanying photos look positively mouthwatering, I noticed that some of the recipes call for ingredients that don't work for me, like PAM cooking spray, white arborio rice, and baby new potatoes. Those items are not on the List. I don't like cooking sprays because many contain alcohol, chemical propellants, or additives, plus the can ends up in the trash. Even so, I highly recommend checking out the website and also reading the print version of the informative *Clean Eating* magazine —

just make slight adjustments to the recipes, like using olive oil from a manual spray pump (or brush) in place of PAM, brown rice instead of arborio, and sweet potatoes rather than new potatoes.

Whatever recipes you choose to prepare at home, make sure your meals have not been made using nonstick (aka Teflon) pans. When nonstick pans reach a high enough temperature, they release toxic chemicals. According to the Environmental Working Group, "This outgassing is sufficiently toxic to kill pet birds and is responsible for 'polymer fume flu' in humans, sometimes called 'Teflon Flu.' Among the symptoms of Teflon Flu are headache, nausea, fever, backache, and malaise." (I had to look up that last word. It's adopted from the French and means discomfort or feeling sick.) Play it safe and ditch your nonstick pans for cast iron, baked enamel, or stainless steel. Whether you call your dinner *clean eating* or simply *chicken enchiladas*, changing the way you look at food to seeing it as fuel and feeling good about what you're putting into your body are critical to your long-term success.

In case you're not completely convinced or if buying only organic foods is simply too costly for you, the Environmental Working Group has created a list of forty-three common fruits and vegetables and ranked them according to pesticide level. And they've even given us the bottom line — the "Dirty Dozen" (the twelve most contaminated items) and the "Cleanest 12" (those that are lowest in pesticides). At a minimum, try your best to always buy the Dirty Dozen fruits and vegetables organic. You can let the items on the "Cleanest 12" list slide if you must. The complete list and a handy downloadable pocket guide are available at www.foodnews.org/walletguide.php. The list may change as conditions change, but here are the current recommendations:

DIRTY DOZEN	CLEANEST TWELVE
1. Peaches	1. Onions
2. Apples	2. Avocados
3. Sweet bell peppers	3. Sweet corn (frozen)
4. Celery	4. Pineapples
5. Nectarines	5. Mangoes
6. Strawberries	6. Sweet peas (frozen)
7. Cherries	7. Asparagus
8. Lettuce	8. Kiwis
9. Imported grapes	9. Bananas
10. Pears	10. Cabbage
11. Spinach	11. Broccoli
12. Potatoes	12. Eggplant

ShopSmart magazine (from the folks at *Consumer Reports*) has some helpful tips on how to eat organic food without breaking the bank. I have modified this list to conserve space and add my own thoughts, but here's the gist of it:

1. SEARCH THE WEB FOR COUPONS.

Stonyfield Farm, Annie's Homegrown, Organic Valley, Earthbound Farm, and Health Valley offer coupons on their websites.

2. BUY IN BULK.

Farmers' markets and many regular grocery stores offer organic items like nuts, grains, cereals, baking supplies, and dried fruit in bulk bins.

3. LOOK FOR STORE-BRAND ORGANICS.

Examples of private-label products are 365 Organic Everyday Value from Whole Foods, Safeway's O Organics, and Trader Joe's, which has literally hundreds of store-brand organic items.

4. JOIN A FOOD CO-OP.

These are run independently and often have a small membership fee, but members get a discount when they shop there. Go to www.coopdirectory.org/directory.htm or www.localharvest .org/food-coops.

5. BUY PRODUCE IN SEASON.

Prices are lowest for fruits and veggies that are in season. To have items year-round, freeze or preserve for later. To see what produce is in season near you, go to www.sustainabletable.org/ shop/eatseasonal.

I've thrown a lot at you here. To simplify, I'll leave you with this before we move on: Make every effort to eat certified-organic food that is in season and grown locally. Buying organic stimulates the demand for more and more farms to use sustainable practices, which makes our drinking water safer and our topsoil healthier. I don't eat 100 percent organic, but I would if it were possible, and I try my very best. The more we all do this, the louder and clearer the message will be conveyed to America's food suppliers.

ITEM #3: ORGANICALLY SPEAKING

1. Try to eat certified-organic foods as often as possible.
2. To improve conditions for workers and growers in developing countries, look for the "Fair Trade" label along with the "Certified Organic" label.
3. Avoid genetically modified organisms (GMOs) by consuming certified-organic foods and looking out for PLU codes on non-certified-organic produce that begin with the number 8.
4. Shop the perimeter of the grocery store, and buy in bulk whenever possible.
5. Don't be duped by confusing terms like *natural* or *contains organic ingredients*.
6. Buy fresher, tastier food that comes from nearby farms and farmers' markets.
7. Eat organic foods that are on the List, and pay close attention to the Environmental Working Group's "Dirty Dozen" and "Cleanest 12."

ITEM #4

FAST FOOD IS FAT FOOD

Truth and Consequences of a Fast-Food Diet

> *Lead me not into temptation;*
> *I can find the way myself.*
> *— Rita Mae Brown*

IF YOU EAT FAST FOOD EVERY DAY or even every other day, take a wild guess why you're overweight. I know it's cheap and convenient, but it's also extremely low quality and full of chemicals, preservatives, and fat. Train yourself to find these foods repulsive. As I mentioned earlier, it will blow your mind to discover how many items at fast-food restaurants contain high fructose corn syrup, from salad dressing to hamburger buns to the applesauce found in kiddy meals.

And how 'bout those patties? Fast-food hamburger meat is made with beef from dozens or even hundreds of different cows. This can lead to a higher chance of contamination because, as Eric Schlosser of *Fast-Food Nation* points out, "If you have one sick cow in the batch, then the risk of getting sick is greater." Because of modern machinery at cattle plants, which scrapes off as much of the meat from the cow as possible, pieces of spinal cord and bone marrow have been discovered in ground beef. This can be extremely dangerous to humans, as spinal cord can transmit mad cow disease. Schlosser's article in *Rolling Stone* magazine shed much-needed light on other ingredients you might find in your fast-food hamburger patty, like the contents of some dead cow's intestine, including fecal matter. Disgusting, to be sure, but this is also a serious matter. Schlosser's article reminds us that while "outbreaks of E. coli have been linked to lettuce, alfalfa sprouts and apple cider, cattle manure has ultimately been the cause of most infections." E. coli found in hamburgers is responsible for deaths occurring each week in this country, as antibiotics do little or nothing to combat this mutated bacteria.

There may be times, such as on long car trips, when fast food seems to be your only option. That's why I'm a big fan of traveling with healthy snacks, like light string cheese, bananas, whole wheat rolls, sliced turkey, and a thermos of water. (Don't forget to use a reusable thermos or metal or glass water bottle as opposed to buying water in plastic bottles, which can pose health risks as well as create a mountain of waste.) Keep yourself satiated, so if you do have to stop for fast food, you won't lose your ability to maintain your good habits. During the previously mentioned, unplanned road trip from Dallas to Amarillo, I didn't have much in the way of snacks, but I did have a bag of raw almonds. I ate nine or ten to keep the hunger pangs at bay.

Even if traffic, road, and weather conditions were okay, I had at least six hours of driving ahead. I would need food. I was prepared for the fact that it wouldn't be organic or meet any of my other criteria for healthy eating. About halfway there, I spotted a Dairy Queen. I hadn't been to a Dairy Queen in years, so I assumed there wouldn't be anything on the List. Much to my delight, there was a grilled chicken salad. I surveyed the list of ingredients and was surprised not to have to make any modifications: chicken, lettuce, tomatoes, carrots, and shredded cheddar cheese. I could always take off some of the cheese if there was too much. There wasn't — cheapskates! I asked for a balsamic vinaigrette dressing, and since it likely contained HFCS, I used only the tiniest amount. After I put the dressing on, I put the lid back on the salad so I could give it a good toss to ensure that each bite would be maximally flavorful. It was a big salad and filled me up enough to get through another three hours of driving.

Other acceptable options for fast food are turkey burgers, grilled chicken sandwiches, and a variety of salads. Remember, white buns are not on the List. Also, skip the croutons, wontons, or tortilla strips, and let me spell it out for you: don't eat the taco salad shell. Some places may even offer a non-cream-based soup. Remember what I said about soup? Soup is your friend.

If you're lucky enough to live in the northwestern United

States, you are likely well acquainted with Burgerville. Burgerville is fast-food perfection. If you live elsewhere, get excited, because I read that the chain was expanding beyond the Pacific Northwest. They use whole grain buns for their turkey burgers, turkey sandwiches, and grilled chicken sandwiches. They also use fresh, seasonal, and local ingredients, buy natural beef from sustainable farms, buy 100 percent renewable wind power for their energy use, pay 95 percent of even their part-time employees' healthcare costs, and convert their used cooking oil to biodiesel. Plus, in 2008, Burgerville started composting in order to reduce waste by 85 percent. That's good news because fast-food restaurants create a massive amount of trash. Composting is a method of dealing with biodegradable waste so it doesn't end up in landfills and create more methane, which is a huge contributor to greenhouse gases. (Composting can be done at home too . . . wink wink, nudge nudge. See www.epa.gov/osw/conserve/rrr/composting for guidelines.)

As far as fast food goes, Burgerville is a company you can feel good about, but stay away from the Walla Walla onion rings and fresh Oregon blackberry milkshakes — so not on the List. I also abstain from the sweet potato fries and bake my own at home. Train yourself to peruse menus and see items as either on the List or not on the List. If you're not sure about an item, assume it's not. Soon this will become second nature to you, and you will make these choices easily and effortlessly and be closer and closer to fitting into your dream pair of jeans.

ITEM #4: FAST FOOD IS FAT FOOD

1. Avoid eating fast food unless you absolutely have to.
2. Take healthy snacks with you on long car rides so you won't be tempted to stop for fast food.
3. If you must eat fast food, avoid milkshakes, anything fried, the low-quality hamburgers, and items containing high fructose corn syrup. Instead, go with a salad, a bowl of non-cream-based soup, or a chicken or turkey burger.
4. If possible, choose places that serve whole wheat buns; otherwise, don't eat the bun.

FAILED ATTEMPTS

IT MAY TAKE THREE OR FOUR REALLY GREAT ATTEMPTS to rid yourself of the soda habit or switch from white to whole wheat sandwich bread. Old habits can be tough to break. Maybe you even have an addiction to food or just to certain foods, like to gummy bears or ice cream — or worse, gummy bears on top of ice cream. If you think your relationship with a particular food is more like an addiction than just a bad habit, get out your calendar. Give up your addiction for twenty-eight days. If you fail, start over. If you fail again, start over. Repeat as needed.

Twenty-eight days is the time frame that rehabilitation centers use to treat drug- and alcohol-addicted patients. If you can refrain for that long, you'll beat your addiction. And what you will learn about yourself in the process is that you are in control. You are not a slave to food or soda pop. You call the shots. You're the boss of you. You — not your body's cravings — decide. Cravings are not trustworthy, but you are. Trust yourself, and know that you are blessed with a powerful mind. Use it to be the best you — one that is on a mission to lose the fat forever — and put your bad habits to rest and replace them with new, healthy, energizing, fat-melting habits that will become second nature so that you will easily and effortlessly make the right choices.

Many people think they are hardwired, that they have little control over their actions and behaviors. Total autopilot. I was chatting with a friend not long ago. He had recently moved into a condo after years of living in a house with a big yard. He said he really likes not having a yard that he "has to" fuss over and be distracted by. He said condo life has freed up a lot of his time because when he had a house and a yard, there was always something to fix or maintain. He said he's the kind of person who can't leave anything undone. If he sees it, he has to tend to it. I say, *Close the blinds*. He said he's hardwired that way and can't help it. Hardwired? You mean just like my sister was hardwired to have a fat ass and not care what she looked like? I say, *It's a choice!* If he wants to spend his days differently, he can make different choices. We aren't robots. We have power and control over our minds and our choices. So read a book, and clean the gutters later. If it's meaningful to you, then change your so-called hardwiring to reflect what you really want. If you truly desire to lose the fat and be slimmer and healthier, then align your habits with what's important to you.

Maybe the way you're wired isn't the problem, and maybe you won't succeed in conquering your addiction for twenty-eight days. Maybe you're one of those people who fails at losing weight because the task seems too overwhelming — you have a considerable amount of fat to lose, and you can't imagine how you'll ever get there. So you give up before you've even started. I say, baby steps. It sounds obvious and terribly cliché, but this approach can work.

A number of years ago, I divorced my children's father. It took me several years to summon the courage to go through with it, and when I finally did, there was no turning back. As a result, I suffered tremendous guilt and went through a period where I could barely get out of bed and function, at least when the kids weren't present. Fortunately, it didn't last very long, but that was because one day as I was lying in bed at eleven in the morning on a school day, I had a thought. I told myself that although I couldn't see beyond one simple task, I could at the very least get up and brush my teeth. It sounds silly and maybe a little more than pathetic, but I got up and brushed my teeth. I then went back to bed until I had to get in the carpool line and pick up the kids. The following day, I not only brushed my teeth; I also took a shower and got dressed. I ended up taking a nap on the couch for the rest of the afternoon, but I was making progress. Those feelings of guilt and sadness were still present, but I was starting to feel better, one small task at a time. Within a month, I was getting out of bed, getting ready for my day, cleaning the house, running errands, and looking for part-time work. Within six months, I was gainfully employed, cochairing the kids' school auction, and hosting dinner parties. It all started with telling myself I could handle one small task — and then actually doing it.

In *Improv Wisdom* by Patricia Ryan Madson, I learned a technique called the "Start Anywhere Rule." When you have a big task ahead and don't know where to begin, start with the most obvious thing or whatever pops into your mind first. Madson explains, "The notion that there is such a thing as a proper beginning, and the search to find the ideal starting place, robs us of time. We distance ourselves from the task, and the vision of what it will take to do it makes tackling the job seem mountainous." Start anywhere. Once you do, you'll be under way. As Madson reminds us, "Once it is under way, any task seems smaller."

So you have some weight to lose, right? Start with one small task — one small habit. You choose what habit you'd like to begin with. Maybe, starting tomorrow, you'll take a half-hour walk in the morning or skip the fast food at lunchtime and make yourself a turkey sandwich and a cup of tomato soup instead. Maybe you'll eat only a small bowl of berries for dessert after dinner.

Whatever new habit you choose to embrace, at the end of the day, take a minute to check in with yourself. Think about how good you feel that you took better care of your body, and imagine what you might add to your efforts the following day or the day after that. One small habit at a time. Once you get rolling, you'll feel an unstoppable amount of momentum, confidence, and accomplishment, and the rest will be history.

MIXERS, MODERATION, AND MARGARITAS

The Big Bottom Line on Booze

*If you are young and you drink a great deal,
it will spoil your health, slow your mind, make you fat —
in other words, turn you into an adult.*
— P. J. O'Rourke

IF YOU'RE LIKE ME and value the medicinal benefits of a glass of red wine and drink only in moderation (I can hear the snickering from my book club pals), what is on the List is pretty simple:

Red and white wines are on the List. Research conducted at the University of Barcelona found that wine, especially red wine, may reduce inflammation in your blood vessels. This could be important because inflammation can lead to the build-up of fatty acids (or plaque) in the walls of your arteries. The *New York Times* has more good news on moderate red wine consumption, reporting that it can help fight obesity as well as slow down aging. If they're available, choose wines that are made from organic grapes, which aren't grown with herbicides, pesticides, and fungicides.

Light beer is on the List. I live in Oregon, the self-proclaimed microbrew capital of America. I like the taste of microbrews, and I feel horrible saying this to all those hard-working, talented brewmasters, but the average microbrew is really fattening! Sorry folks, but microbrews are not on the List.

Hard alcohol by itself or with club soda or water is on the List. I like to keep it simple, but if you'd like to spice things up a bit, add a splash of unsweetened cranberry juice. This adds next to nothing in the way of calories or sugar, and pure, 100 percent cranberry juice is rich in antioxidants and may lower bad cholesterol. According to Ann Louise Gittleman of *The Fat Flush Plan*, cranberries are reported to have properties that promote weight loss. She writes, "Cranberry juice contains high levels of organic acids, which have an emulsifying effect upon fat deposits." Hard alcohol is more concentrated and therefore can be tougher on your filtering organs, so be kind to your body and opt for water, wine, or light beer more often than hard alcohol.

So what's not on the List? Cocktails and mixed drinks. One cocktail can have upward of six or seven hundred calories. A typical margarita or piña colada can easily have around five hundred calories — compared to a vodka soda, which has considerably less, at one hundred calories, and contains zero sugar. Sweet and fruity cocktails are mostly sugar, fruit juice, and premade mixers that are mostly high fructose corn syrup. They can make you fat. Cocktails are not on the List.

ITEM #5: MIXERS, MODERATION, AND MARGARITAS

Before you get too excited and think you have the green light on drinking wine, light beer, and hard alcohol, we should chat about what is considered moderate drinking. Consuming more than a glass or two a day even just a few days per week will likely pack on the pounds and may adversely affect your health. (Exception: If you're in Italy, drink wine with every meal. Drink wine all day if you want. On second thought, don't do that — you might do something stupid and then blame me for your behavior.)

The Harvard School of Public Health's website says drinking alcohol is a balancing act. It states, "If you are thin, physically active, don't smoke, eat a healthy diet, and have no family history of heart disease, drinking alcohol won't add much to decreasing your risk of cardiovascular disease." They also say to keep it moderate; no more than two drinks a day for men or one drink a day for women.

To slow down the absorption of alcohol, eat while you drink — or eat before you drink. Good choices are whole grain carbs and light protein snacks like whole wheat crackers, raw almonds, a small handful of olives, or a small bowl of whole grain cereal. I'm not telling you something you don't already know, but alcohol greatly reduces your ability to make good choices. I know this for a fact. My dad explained it to me in far too graphic detail when I was young because I asked why I had to have little brothers. Once I've had a few too many, the List goes out the window and I wind up eating a basket of fries or an entire pepperoni pizza. Ease up on the alcohol to avoid eating excessively or eating junk food while drinking.

Overeating and hangovers not excluded, there are plenty of other physiological reasons to avoid overdoing it with alcohol, including liver damage, reproductive problems, and interference with prescription medications. Those are all superb reasons to limit your alcohol consumption, but getting fat and having premature wrinkles and excessive cellulite speak pretty darn loudly to me as well.

Make a plan to wean yourself from overindulging in alcohol. Let's say you're a wine drinker and drink a few glasses every night. You're consuming roughly three hundred extra calories a day with that seemingly moderate habit. In a week, you're consuming about twenty or more glasses, which could easily translate to an additional one- or two-pound weight gain each week — or weight loss if you kicked this habit. What if you consumed only one bottle (750 ml) of wine, which contains approximately five five-ounce glasses, spread out over a week? This would dramatically decrease your wine consumption and still allow you to enjoy your favorite wines. Another idea that is a bit more restrictive is to drink only on special occasions. You may want to clearly define what "special occasion" means to you. In my book, watching television doesn't qualify. Cutting back is the key. If you enjoy one glass of wine while preparing dinner and then another while eating dinner, decide which one has to go; then let it go. Make it a habit, and you are one step closer to having the healthy body you want.

ITEM #5: MIXERS, MODERATION, AND MARGARITAS

(...for those of legal age and who choose to consume alcohol)

1. Choose white or red wine, light beer, or hard alcohol (straight, with water, or with club soda).
2. Look for organic wines that don't contain herbicides, pesticides, and fungicides.
3. Avoid cocktails and mixed drinks.
4. Drink moderately: no more than one or two drinks a day, and only a few days per week.

ITEM #6

FOO-FOO COFFEE DRINKS

The Skinny on Caffeinated Beverages

> *Call things what they are.*
> *If your morning coffee contains*
> *crushed ice, whipped cream, and caramel,*
> *it's a milkshake!*
> *— Bill Maher*

'LL TAKE A DECAF SUGAR-FREE TRIPLE GRANDE two-pump mocha with whip please." Sound familiar? Sorry for the buzz-kill, but foo-foo coffee drinks like mochas, flavored lattes, and Frappuccinos can make you fat. If your coffee comes with a clear plastic domed lid, it's time to rethink your drink order. Switch to tea, coffee, a nonfat café au lait, or a nonfat latte. Add a tiny amount of raw brown sugar or honey if you need a little sweetener. Agave nectar and stevia, mentioned in Item #1, are other natural choices for sweeteners. I've found that milk already has a sweet taste and I rarely need to add anything to my café au laits or lattes. For regular coffee, skim milk is better, but half-and-half or real cream in extremely small doses is on the List. Packaged coffee creamers and powdered creamers are typically chock-full of corn syrup, trans fats (aka partially hydrogenated oils, which we'll be discussing later), chemicals, and unnecessary "fake" ingredients. They are not on the List, end of story. Consume real food.

Tea is a superb choice: it has no calories, much less caffeine than coffee, and a load of medicinal benefits, and certain types are reported to rev up your metabolism. Antioxidant-rich green tea is the real superstar (more on antioxidants in Item #9). Green, black, and oolong tea all come from the *Camellia sinensis* plant, but only the green tea leaves are steamed, leaving them unfermented so they don't become oxidized. That's a complicated way of saying that all the medicinal properties are left intact and you get the biggest boost to your health, with possible benefits including cancer prevention, a decrease in rheumatoid arthritis symptoms, reversal of sun damage, lower cholesterol, a reduced risk of heart disease, and improved immune function. A study at Purdue University says adding a squeeze of lemon juice to your green tea increases the chances of those antioxidants surviving the digestive process by five times.

I have a cup of hot green tea along with my midmorning snack, which is typically one piece of light string cheese and a small handful of raw almonds or walnuts. Any later in the day, and the caffeine in the tea would keep me up at night, and I love my sleep. Did you know that getting plenty of sleep could help you maintain your optimum metabolism? According to a study conducted by two Northwestern University researchers and published in the *Archives of Internal Medicine*, a lack of sleep can make you fat. They studied how "loss of sleep alters the complex metabolic pathways that control appetite, food intake, and energy expenditure." I truly believe that sleep matters. I've been going to sleep embarrassingly early my entire life, and I think I have a pretty kickass metabolism. So try your best to get your eight hours in. Research in the journal *Cell Metabolism* found that cutting out saturated fats and trans fats may be a way to improve your sleep and help control late-night snacking — it worked for a bunch of mice, anyway.

The next time you go to Starbucks (or better yet, a locally owned coffeehouse that serves organic, fair-trade coffee), whether you opt for tea, coffee, or a nonfat café au lait, when the barista asks, "Would you care for a pastry to go with your coffee today?" answer her with, "No, thank you. I don't eat white, fattening, sugar-filled, fake, high–glycemic index foods anymore. I used to, but now I make good choices because I want to be slender and healthy and bursting with energy." Don't be afraid to speak your mind. Your barista will enjoy getting to know you better. Take her giant eye roll to mean that she truly appreciates where you're coming from. You may have guessed where I'm coming from — pastries are not on the List. Some Starbucks (and the like) offer whole grain sandwiches and breakfast bars, oatmeal, and an assortment of salads. I don't trust anything without a label, and I'm not about to make a big fuss when there are a half dozen people in line, so if I can't readily see what's in it, I don't order it. When I'm out shopping for wardrobe items for a TV commercial and Starbucks is the only available lunch option, the turkey club sandwich on whole grain bread, minus the cheese, bacon, and mayo, is a high-protein, lowfat choice and is far better than the egg or tuna salad sandwich, which are both made with mayonnaise and consequently much higher in fat and calories.

With Starbucks stores closing all over the country, maybe this is pointless advice, but at least for the time being, Portland has a Starbucks on nearly every block. Unless I'm on a job, I rarely set foot in any of them. In Portland, those in the know are loyal to Stumptown Coffee, which is vastly superior to any other coffee. Unfortunately, though, as much as I love the beautiful nature designs they make with the foam on my latte, I can't patronize them during the week because the line is a mile long and the artistic drink execution sucks up half my morning. I stop by on the weekend, pick up some organic, fair-trade beans, and brew my coffee at home. I take it with skim milk or, on occasion, a teaspoon of real half-and-half and a tiny amount of raw brown sugar or agave nectar. Whether you make coffee at home or stop by a local café every morning before work, train yourself to order only what's on the List and decline the pastry offer.

Debate abounds on whether drinking coffee is a good idea. I've read countless articles containing all sorts of conflicting evidence about the good and the bad of drinking coffee.

ITEM #6: FOO-FOO COFFEE DRINKS

What scares me the most is the link between caffeine and osteoporosis (or the weakening of the bones), which can lead to fractures or broken hips. Granted, they were all well into their eighties or nineties when they died, but every one of my great aunts was hunched over and looking down at her shoes for the last ten years of her life. To be good to your bones, you need calcium.

The Mayo Clinic website cautions that excessive amounts of caffeine can rob your body of calcium and lead to osteoporosis. The good news is they say that for most people, moderate coffee drinking is considered around two or three cups a day. I can live with that. Dr. Mehmet Oz of the *YOU* book series is okay with up to twenty-four ounces of daily coffee. He also says that coffee is America's largest source of antioxidants and, "Studies consistently show that coffee and caffeine reduce the risk of Parkinson's, and may even protect against Alzheimer's disease and cancer." Moreover, I read in *Parade* magazine recently that drinking coffee is one of the top ways to ensure that you live to triple digits.

On the flip side — because, darn it, there always is one — coffee may contribute to your being overweight. I've managed to stay thin while drinking coffee so far, but coffee may increase your levels of a stress hormone called cortisol, which can increase your appetite and cause a loss of muscle mass. I know that green tea may be the better choice, and I make sure to drink a monster mug of it every day, but first thing in the morning, I'm sticking with my antioxidant-rich cup o' joe — the daily paper wouldn't be the same without it.

ITEM #6: FOO-FOO COFFEE DRINKS

1. Eliminate foo-foo coffee drinks from your life.
2. Order coffee, tea, or a nonfat latte or café au lait, and sweeten it with one teaspoon of raw brown sugar, raw honey, or an alternative sweetener like agave nectar or stevia.
3. Do not use packaged creamers; stick with nonfat milk (best choice) or a dollop of half-and-half or cream.
4. Get a good night's sleep to keep your metabolism at its peak.
5. Pass over the pastries at coffee shops, and eat breakfast at home.

THE MOST IMPORTANT MEAL OF THE DAY

Break the Fast to Shed Pounds, Boost Metabolism, and Prevent Overeating

> *It is never too late to be what you might have been.*
> — *George Eliot*

TO MAINTAIN OPTIMUM METABOLISM, you absolutely, positively need a good breakfast. Many fat people and constant dieters skip breakfast. They're trying to be good and limit their daily intake of calories, but their metabolism takes a nosedive, and they end up with an unstoppable appetite and make bad choices for the rest of the day. Your basal metabolism, measured as your basal metabolic rate (BMR), is the rate at which your body burns energy, in the form of calories, while it is at rest. The faster your metabolism is, the more efficiently your body burns fat. Credit for part of the clever chapter subtitle goes to WebMD.com, which says, "Break the fast to shed the pounds. Overweight and obese children, adolescents, and adults are less likely to break the fast each morning than their thinner counterparts."

The way to jump-start your metabolism is to eat in the morning! To get my metabolism going, I eat as soon as I wake up. Unless I have the flu or a six a.m. flight, I don't skip breakfast. I also make good choices. You can have pancakes, waffles, or French toast as long as they are whole grain and you go easy on the portions and the butter and syrup. Use real maple syrup and not fake or lite syrup, which contains high fructose corn syrup. Maple syrup packs a lot of taste in a small amount, so use as little as possible. I use real butter, but too much butter can add a lot of unhealthy, saturated fat to your otherwise hale and hearty breakfast. I don't normally go for pancakes or waffles, but mostly because I'm too lazy to make them or clean up the mess. I prefer a bowl of oatmeal, an omelet or a scramble (with mostly egg whites; more on this below) with chicken-apple sausage, or a bowl of plain nonfat yogurt sweetened with agave nectar with fresh berries and a few chopped raw almonds on top.

Be cautious with cereal. Foods in boxes and other packages can contain some risky ingredients, like white sugar, high fructose corn syrup, trans fats (see Item #10), GMOs, and preservatives. I opt for organic whole grain cereals that contain fiber and protein and as few ingredients as possible. I eat my cereal with nonfat milk or plain nonfat yogurt. Thanks to stores like Trader Joe's, Whole Foods, New Seasons, Henry's, and Greenwise, many cereals meet my criteria. Smaller, local stores that sell organic foods are great places to find decent options as well.

I feel like I haven't talked enough about my total and complete enthusiasm for eggs. I call it "eggthusiasm." (If you haven't figured it out by now, I'm a dork. I can be a snazzy dresser, though, so you wouldn't know it just by looking at me.) I like my eggs scrambled, poached, boiled, or made into an omelet.

Mind you, not all egg dishes are created equal. Quiches and frittatas aren't a great choice. Quiche has a pie crust that is loaded with calories, fat, and sometimes sugar. If you make sure to remove the entire crust or make the quiche yourself with whole wheat flour and very little cheese and load it with vegetables and an optional lean meat, then go ahead and have a slice. Frittatas are often made with eggs and chunks of potatoes. Hold the potatoes or substitute sweet potatoes, and they deserve a spot on the List. Then there's eggs Benedict, about the worst choice you can make when dining out for breakfast (followed by chicken fried steak, steak and eggs, Belgian waffles, and corned beef hash). A typical order of eggs Benedict has roughly eighty grams of fat, very little fiber, and a whopping nine hundred calories — and that's before the side of hash browns, glass of o.j., and double mocha.

I'll share a little secret with you. You can eat a giant plate of eggs if you use mostly egg whites. Fewer egg yolks cut down on the fat, calories, and cholesterol and actually make for fluffier omelets and scrambles. Load 'em up with a bunch of sautéed veggies, black beans, a touch of Parmesan cheese, and slices of chicken-apple sausage. My scrambles are obscenely big, and I eat every bite, guilt free. I cook my scrambles in olive oil because I like the flavor and because olive oil contains the good type of fat my body needs. Eggs are at the top of the List.

What about milk? Does it do a body good? Eating dairy is yet another topic that creates heated debates, and we are left not knowing if we should trust the government, the dairy industry, or the growing anti-dairy movement that claims that cow's milk is only for baby cows. (I know they're really called calves, but "baby cows" sounds so much cuter.) Even the beloved and trusted pediatrician Dr. Spock jumped on the anti-dairy bandwagon before his death. Folks in the anti-dairy camp say the only time we should be drinking milk is when we are babies, and that milk should come from our mothers. Some say that drinking milk creates mucus and our body reacts by developing allergies to ward off the alien substance. And what about dairy cows being fed antibiotics and hormones, which may be contributing to girls starting menstruation at an increasingly earlier age? Just another reason to buy certified-organic foods for you and your family as often as possible.

On the other side of the discussion, the dairy industry and the food pyramid created by the dieticians at the United States Department of Agriculture say we need dairy products as part of a healthy, balanced diet. So should we be eating milk, cheese, butter, and yogurt, or not? The Harvard School of Public Health presents a balanced view on the Nutrition page of its website. It states four reasons why milk and other dairy products may not be a good source of calcium for some. Those suffering from lactose intolerance will obviously need to find another source, but aside from that, dairy products have been linked to heart disease and a possible increased risk of ovarian and prostate cancers. For people not predisposed to these conditions, lowfat or nonfat dairy products are recommended, but the website points out that there are other good sources of calcium, like dark green leafy vegetables, beans and other legumes, oranges, almonds, and green peas. It recommends a daily consumption of 1,000 milligrams for those fifty and under, and 1,200 milligrams for those over fifty. To put that in perspective, a one-cup serving of cooked collard greens contains 350 milligrams. I wish you tremendous luck getting your four-year-old to eat a serving of collard greens.

Eating fortified dairy products helps make sure you're also getting some vitamin D, which aids in the absorption of calcium and the prevention of osteoporosis, prostate cancer, breast cancer, and even obesity. It also eases depression and the effects of diabetes. In one of his regular monthly articles in *Esquire* magazine, Dr. Oz says vitamin D also helps reduce the risk of immune disorders and heart disease. But fortified dairy is not the only way to get your daily dose of vitamin D. I also try to get fifteen or twenty minutes of natural sunlight every day, but I take precautions so that it's absorbed through the skin on my limbs and not on my face, where I'm more susceptible to skin cancer and premature wrinkles. Sunblock and a hat help with that potential hazard. My dermatologist used to say shun the sun and take a vitamin D supplement instead, but now she advises minimal daily sun exposure for low-risk individuals and being careful to protect high-risk skin areas like the face and neck. Vitamin D is getting a lot of press lately because doctors are finding that more and more of their patients are deficient in it. Michael Holick, MD, author of *The UV Advantage*, exposes some of the myths circulating about vitamin D in an interview reported on Naturalnews.com. He says that sun exposure is the only reliable way to get adequate amounts of vitamin D and that sitting in your car or next to a window in your home or office won't work because the beneficial effects of sunlight are not transmitted through glass.

I eat dairy. I drink very little milk and when I do, it's non-fat or lowfat. I eat light string cheese, lowfat sour cream, and nonfat or lowfat yogurt (always certified organic, of course). Real yogurt contains probiotics, which, at least to me, sound disgusting because they're bacteria, but they're the good kind of bacteria that help maintain a proper balance of healthy flora in your intestinal tract. I just eat it and don't think about the legions of necessary bacteria that are lurking inside my body at all times. According to a study published in *Molecular Systems Biology*, probiotics can also improve metabolism and digestion and promote weight loss. With the exception of the occasional teaspoon of cream I add to my coffee and the even rarer teaspoon of real butter I slather on my whole grain toast, I don't consume high-fat dairy products in the form of milk, cheese, or ice cream. I'd be bummed if I had to give up dairy, but I also don't seem to have developed any problems related to consuming it.

I maintain the same balanced view of dairy that is presented by the brainiacs at the Harvard School of Public Health. The jury is still out, and there is much in the way of conflicting information. I'm not overweight and I eat dairy, but always in moderation and always with as little fat as possible. There are tons of dairy substitutes available, and some are List-approved, like unsweetened organic soy milk and rice milk. I'm not big on substitutes, but if it ever becomes abundantly clear that I am damaging my health by eating dairy, I may give them a try. Do what makes sense for you.

Just so we're clear on this breakfast business: No white foods. No pastries or muffins. No scones. No sugary cereals. No hash browns or cottage fries. And no juice.

At least, I don't drink juice. There could be some arguments for drinking real 100 percent fruit juice. Pomegranate juice is loaded with antioxidants and is supposedly good for men's prostate health. Lemonade has been shown to slow the development of painful kidney stones. A high concentration of cranberry juice keeps bacteria from sticking to the bladder wall and can prevent urinary tract infections. To me, though, juice means extra calories. I'd rather have a piece of fruit that contains half the calories but also has bulk and fills me up. I eat fruit throughout the day, but I make sure to start every day with a piece of fruit. Most fruit is low on the glycemic index, which means it's a good carb, but fruit is also chock-full of important enzymes, vitamins, and minerals and is the perfect sweet treat.

I'm not a proponent of smoothies — especially at juice bars. Smoothies can be high in calories and sugar and are often used as meal replacements, but does that ever work? I'm always starving an hour after I drink a smoothie, but I've put away upward of four hundred calories, making it hard to justify eating anything else until the next mealtime. Those of you making the concoctions yourself and mostly from veggies or real fruit have the green light, but personally, I need food that I can eat, that has substance, and that will keep me satiated.

What? No juice? No hash browns? No buttery scones? Nope. Not on the List. Remember, you have control over your mind. So change it. Think of these foods as foods that you don't eat. Period. Think whole grain, good; white and starchy, bad. Think green tea good; foo-foo latte milkshakes, bad. Remember to break the fast and fuel your body up first thing in the morning. Treat yourself kindly, and make the time to fix yourself a healthy and delicious scramble or bowl of oatmeal with brown sugar or agave nectar, blueberries, and raw almonds. Train yourself to see food differently, and it will become a habit — a habit that can help melt away the fat easily and effortlessly.

ITEM #7: THE MOST IMPORTANT MEAL OF THE DAY

1. Eat breakfast every morning.
2. Eat whole grain pancakes, waffles, and French toast with real maple syrup.
3. Use half egg whites in your scrambles and omelets.
4. Eat nonfat or lowfat yogurt with berries and nuts.
5. Avoid pastries as well as packaged foods with white sugar, trans fats, or high fructose corn syrup.
6. Ditch the hash browns or substitute sweet potatoes.
7. Try dairy substitutes if you have problems associated with eating dairy products or worry that it may lead to heart disease or other ailments.
8. Eat fruit with your breakfast, but limit juices and avoid high-calorie smoothies. Drink water, tea, or coffee.

GOING TO EXTREMES

I HAVE A STORY FOR YOU ABOUT ANOTHER FRIEND — one of my closest friends. I'll call her "Stupid." Calling her that makes me appear horribly unkind, but I think she'd prefer it over my revealing her real name. Plus, I think you'll agree that it's a fitting term after reading this. Stupid lost a bunch of weight last year. According to Stupid, she has yo-yo dieted too many times over the years and has compromised her metabolism, so the only way for her to lose weight is to go to extremes. Research at the Indiana University School of Medicine indicates that the idea that yo-yo dieting compromises your metabolism is a myth and that it is absolutely possible to retrain your metabolism. The *American Journal of Clinical Nutrition* found the same to be true in its 1992 study. Stupid claimed, however, that the only way for her to lose weight was by not eating or only eating one tiny meal a day.

She did lose the fat, and fast, but she also ended up in the hospital. She called me from work one day crying because she had tunnel vision and was seeing waves and feeling extremely lightheaded. I told her to eat something. She started crying even harder. She thought she needed to go to the emergency room. I thought she needed to go to the café across the street and eat some toast — some whole grain toast. She agreed to eat a little something, and I agreed to pick her up and take her to the emergency room. The intake nurse asked her a series of questions, all of which Stupid answered with total lies. She answered no when asked if anything unusual had taken place recently. Dramatic weight loss achieved by starving yourself is likely worth mentioning. Since Stupid wouldn't tell the truth, I did it for her. The nurse began vigorously taking notes.

On the way to the hospital, Stupid had told me that during the prior forty-eight-hour period, she had eaten only one small salad. That's it! I had to bust her. Stupid knows how serious starving yourself is — both her aunt and her cousin died of anorexia! Now do you see why I call her Stupid? When we got in to see the doctor (Stupid told them I was her sister), she repeated the same lies all over again. When I gave her the look that said, "I'm going to tell her or you are," she made a half-assed attempt at the truth, but Stupid wasn't taking any of it seriously. She was in total denial. Fortunately, the ER doc saw right through Stupid's story and gave her a stern lecture about the risks of starvation dieting.

Starvation dieting will compromise your metabolism and can actually lead to weight gain. But more important, it can put you at risk for serious health problems and in some cases can cause death. The Mayo Clinic's website describes the types of crazy and dangerous things that can happen to our bodies when we don't eat or when we don't eat enough; the most severe cases are people with anorexia nervosa. Those with this disease are obsessed with food, weight, and body shape, so they starve themselves. This can cause abnormal heart rhythms and heart failure, bone loss, lung problems, the absence of menstrual periods in women, decreased testosterone in men, constipation, bloating, nausea, electrolyte abnormalities, kidney problems, and death. The Mayo Clinic warns, "If a person with anorexia becomes severely malnourished, every organ in the body can sustain damage, including the brain, heart, and kidneys. This damage may not be fully reversible, even when the anorexia is under control." Those are just the physiological problems. The mental problems include depression, anxiety disorders, personality disorders, obsessive-compulsive disorders, and addiction.

If it takes a little while to reach your ideal, healthy weight, then that's what it takes. The point is not to end up in the hospital. You are not in a fat-burning race. There is no quick fix, and when you don't take the time to lose weight with habits you can sustain over the long run, the weight will inevitably return.

I had a conversation with another friend about her lifelong battle with obesity. I don't know her well enough to give her a harsh name like Stupid, but she shared with me that she'd recently lost ten to twelve pounds on the Atkins diet. This discussion took place during a weekend trip with a group of friends. At first I just listened and observed. When we went out for breakfast, she ordered a cheese-laden omelet and a side of bacon. Before dinner one night, she ate tons of vegetables but also munched on handfuls of smoked nuts and cubes of cheese. At dinner, she downed a hefty steak. At a Starbucks stop, she took four packets of Equal in her ice tea. This gal is considerably overweight and was recently diagnosed with type 2 diabetes and now requires medication, which, at the young age of thirty-seven, she finds quite unsettling. She said she used to eat white carbs by the truckload, which could have led to her diabetic condition. On day two of our trip, after I'd enjoyed a few glasses of wine (it was a special occasion), I saddled up next to her in a window seat for a little girl chat. She's more of a friend of a friend and someone I wanted to get to know better, so I tried a delicate approach rather than my usual bulldozer style. I blame the wine, because that subtle tactic did not last long.

I commended her for trying to get control of her weight. I also told her that I was concerned with a few aspects of her diet, specifically the large amounts of saturated fat and sodium, the artificial sweeteners, and the sheer number of calories she was eating. She said she'd never felt better and was extremely pleased with her progress. I shared with her my findings from the *Journal of Commonsense Eating* and did my best to convince her that in the long run, that weight will return and there could be serious and harmful consequences from a diet high in saturated fat and sodium. I forgot to mention that, in the meantime, her breath would smell like a litter box and she would spend most of her days constipated. She said she's the kind of person who needs quick results and her new diet was working. I understand her eagerness to lose weight as well as her strong desire to get off medication, but I fervently challenged her to recall one time in her life when anything beneficial, meaningful, or long-lasting happened as a result of taking a shortcut.

Unfortunately, I wasn't able to persuade her that eating whole grain, high-fiber, low-glycemic carbs is the path to permanent, albeit slower, weight loss. I did plead with her to make a few modifications in the interest of her health: eat lean meats and only the occasional serving of red meat or bacon; ease up on the cubes of cheese and handfuls of salty, smoked nuts; and discontinue using Equal or other fake sugars, since she was not on doctor's order to do so. She probably just wanted the conversation to come to a crashing halt, but she agreed. I wrapped up my lengthy rant by telling her I would send her a copy of my book so that if the weight came back, she could read it.

This type of extreme dieting is next to impossible to maintain, so even though you've had some success losing weight, you've compromised your health and you can all but count on seeing that weight come back in the future. Celebrate the modest progress you achieve every day by eating well, drinking plenty of water, getting much-needed exercise, and changing your habits so today's extra weight will one day be history and not a part of your future.

When my sister lost considerable weight over a nine-month period, she didn't think about how many pounds she was losing per week. In fact, she didn't set any weight-loss goals at all.

She changed her habits and how she looked at food and saw it as a new, lifelong way of healthy living. She saw that good things were happening because her clothes were getting looser by the week, her energy level was increasing tenfold, and her knees, back, and feet weren't aching as often. Now, Stupid is a whole other story, and I'm still keeping an eye on her because I love her dearly and want her to live. Please don't be like Stupid, okay?

ITEM #8

MEAT ME IN THE MIDDLE

A Balanced Approach to Healthful
and Ethical Meat Consumption

It is unwise to be too sure of one's own wisdom.
It is healthy to be reminded that the strongest
might weaken and the wisest might err.
— Mohandas Gandhi

A S YOU'VE LIKELY FIGURED OUT BY NOW, I eat animal meat.
However, there are countless reasons why eating meat is
not such a great idea. There are moral and ethical reasons, reli-
gious reasons, environmental reasons, and health reasons. I am
fairly defenseless in justifying my consumption of animal meat.
I once gave it up for almost three years. I'd like to say it was for
ethical reasons, but truthfully, I just got temporarily grossed out
by it. Then one day I had the most intense craving for a turkey
sandwich, and that was it. Because we love our labels, the term
ethical omnivores has been given to meat eaters and dairy eaters
who pursue their love of meat and dairy wholeheartedly but
only if the animals are raised in humane conditions.

Plant-based foods are significantly more efficient to produce than animal-based foods, so I do my best to balance my enthusiasm for meat by consciously making an effort to eat other protein sources, like heart-healthy legumes, whenever possible. They are high in fiber, low on the glycemic index, and low in fat, sodium, and calories. And don't forget nuts and seeds. Lightly toasted, robust, dense breads made with nuts and seeds are incredibly satisfying. Throw a couple of poached eggs on top, and I'm a happy girl.

Getting your protein from sources other than beef is a pretty brilliant idea. An article in *Domino* magazine says, "If 10,000 people gave up steak once every seven days, it'd conserve enough water annually to fill 22,719 Olympic-size swimming pools." That image provides a pretty astounding picture of just how resource-intensive beef production is. On top of that, the U.S. Environmental Protection Agency estimates that nearly 75 percent of the water pollution in the United States is a direct result of industrial beef production and processing. The problems associated with global warming and climate change are also increased due to beef production and consumption: cows emit enormous amounts of methane, a potent greenhouse gas. (As difficult as it is to show some restraint here, I will not be making a smartass comment about farting. I may be a dork, but I'm not a twelve-year-old boy.)

Also, decomposing manure releases large quantities of nitrous oxide, an air pollutant that produces acid rain and can put humans at risk for respiratory illnesses. In addition, the *New York Times* reports, "about two to five times more grain is required to produce the same amount of calories through livestock as through direct grain consumption, according to Rosamond Naylor, an associate professor of economics at Stanford University. It is as much as 10 times more in the case of grain-fed beef in the United States." This results in an ever-increasing amount of land used to grow livestock feed instead of food for human consumption. Frances Moore Lappé, author of *Diet for a Small Planet*, asks us to imagine sitting down to an eight-ounce steak. "Then," she writes, "imagine the room filled with forty-five to fifty people with empty bowls in front of them. For the 'feed cost' of your steak, each of their bowls could be filled with a full cup of cooked cereal grains."

From a health standpoint, there are many reasons to limit your beef consumption. Beef is a leading source of dietary saturated fat, which can significantly increase the risk of heart disease. Some studies suggest that excessive meat consumption can also increase the risk of certain cancers and may contribute to the formation of kidney stones. Beef consumption also creates a significant number of public health hazards. Animal feed in industrial meat plants may contain arsenic, animal by-products, and antibiotics. The routine use of antibiotics in cattle feed has contributed to the development of antibiotic-resistant strains of common pathogens like staphylococcus (you know, the stuff that causes staph infections) and tuberculosis. Equally frightening, animal by-products that are added to the food of livestock contribute to the spread of mad cow disease.

If you're like me and choose to eat animal meat along with

other great sources of protein like lentils, beans, nuts, seeds, and dairy, try to eat lean meats like chicken, turkey, bison (aka buffalo) more often than fattier ones like pork, lamb, and beef. It's also critical to eat high-quality meat that doesn't contain antibiotics or growth hormones. Certified-organic meat is guaranteed to be free of those things, but when purchasing beef, also look for the label "Grass Fed." Feeding cattle grass instead of grain makes the meat healthier because it contains more omega-3 fatty acids than grain-fed beef and contains less fat overall — not only less fat, but less saturated fat, which contributes to cardiovascular disease and other health problems. Game animals like bison eat only grass; they would get sick otherwise. According to the USDA, bison has less than half the fat of chicken and one-third the fat of pork. The bad news is that it's hard to find. Finding a local butcher who sells it would be your best bet; otherwise, you can order it online. Two popular sources are Northforkbison.com and Healthybuffalo.com.

Maybe this isn't obvious to you, but if you see fat on your meat, don't eat it. Cut it off and move it to the side of your plate. I eat pretty large portions of the lean meats and pretty small portions of the fattier meats. When I eat meat, I also eat a lot of vegetables. I tend to get my whole grains at breakfast and lunch, so my dinner plate is usually two-thirds veggies and one-third protein, which for me consists of animal meat, seafood, soy, or legumes. Go easy on sauces. The fat and calories in gravy and white sauces can do a lot of damage to an otherwise healthy, low-fat plateful.

Did you happen to catch that I just snuck "soy" in that list of proteins? Soy is a tricky one. Most soy-based meat substitutes are heavily processed, and the ones that are not certified organic will likely contain genetically modified soybeans. Every once in a while, especially if I'm at a burger joint that doesn't claim or cannot confirm that their beef is grass fed, free of hormones and antibiotics, and raised using sustainable practices, I go for the veggie burger or soy burger. To me, neither is an ideal choice, but I feel safer having an overly processed, possibly GMO-laced, plant-based food than something that might give me mad cow disease or E. coli and, well, kill me. I'm cutting my losses, so to speak. At least, tofu and tempeh, both soy-based, are closer to a more natural, whole form. And the vegetable and brown rice–based Gardenburger? Their "original" patty has thirty-eight ingredients! That alone makes me suspicious.

Eating fish also poses a conundrum. On the one hand, you've got the extremely healthy aspects of fish: fish is high in protein and low in fat, and many varieties have a high concentration of essential omega-3 fatty acids, which help maintain good cardiovascular health. A Harvard School of Public Health study shows that eating a modest amount of fish (about 3 ounces of farmed salmon or 6 ounces of mackerel) every week reduces the risk of death from coronary heart disease by 36 percent and overall mortality (deaths from any cause) by 17 percent.

Those are pretty impressive numbers, so what's the problem? High levels of toxins such as mercury, to start with. Throw in the fact that marine habitats are being destroyed at an alarming rate, and what's a fish lover to do? First of all, pay attention to how the fish you're buying was caught and where it was caught. The Environmental Defense Organization (EDO) says that high-impact fishing methods often kill dolphins, seals, and whales in the process of catching fish and that fish-farming practices are good for some seafood types but create a problematic situation for others.

Farmed salmon, for example, are raised in such tight quarters that sea lice spread quickly and can also affect wild fish swimming nearby. Because of this, antibiotics, parasiticides, and other chemicals that can pollute and contaminate surrounding waters are often used. The EDO explains that farmed oysters, clams, and bay scallops, on the other hand, are raised on suspension nets, so they have a lower impact on ocean habitat, since dredging, which can damage the seafloor, is not necessary to harvest them.

A quick and easy way to determine if a specific fish is healthy for you *and* for ocean habitats is to get out your cell phone and text *30644* and type *fish* and the name of the fish you're interested in. Seafoodwatch.org will send you a return text message and let you know if you're in the clear. If you have a little more time, the EDO has established criteria for "Eco-Best" seafood, which it defines as "wild fish caught from healthy, well-managed populations using low-impact fishing gear; or farmed fish raised in systems that control pollution, chemical use and escapes." Good news for us fish lovers: it's a pretty long list. To sort it out by fish type, check the EDO's website often because as conditions change, so does the list. The site also lists "Eco-OK" and "Eco-Worst" seafood and even has a handy pocket guide you can print out. The list is available at Edf.org. As of this writing, the current list of "Eco-Best" is as follows:

Abalone

Anchovies

Barramundi

Catfish (U.S.)

Caviar (farmed)

Char, Arctic (farmed)

Clams (farmed)

Clams, softshell

Cod, Pacific (longline)

Crab, Dungeness

Crab, stone

Crawfish (U.S.)

Halibut, Pacific

Lobster, California spiny

Lobster, Caribbean spiny
   (U.S.)

Mackerel, Atlantic

Mahimahi (U.S. troll/pole)

Mullet

Mussels

Oysters (farmed)

Paddlefish (farmed)

Pollock, Alaska (U.S.)

Prawn spot (Canada)

Sablefish (Alaska, Canada)

Salmon, canned

Salmon, wild (Alaska)

Sardines, Pacific (U.S.)

Scallops, bay (farmed)

Shrimp, pink (Oregon)

Shrimp (U.S. farmed)

Squid, longfin (U.S.)

Striped bass (farmed)

Sturgeon, white (farmed)

Tilapia (U.S.)

Trout, rainbow (farmed)

Tuna, albacore (U.S., Canada)

Tuna, yellowfin (U.S.
   Atlantic troll/pole)

Wreckfish

Like I've said, I keep it simple. When it comes to eating meat, I pretty much stick with "Eco-Best" seafood or organic, free-range chicken breast and call it good. I'm certainly no vegan, but those at Goveg.com say, "chickens on today's factory farms almost always become crippled because their legs cannot support the weight of their bodies. In fact, by the age of 6 weeks, 90 percent of broiler chickens are so obese that they can no longer walk." Support chicken suppliers that maintain compassionate living conditions and sell only organic, free-range chicken raised without antibiotics and hormones. Being an ethical omnivore is good for you, the animals, and the planet.

ITEM #8: MEAT ME IN THE MIDDLE

1. Eat heart-healthy beans, legumes, seeds, and nuts as a regular source of protein.
2. Eat lean meats like chicken, fish, and buffalo more often than beef, lamb, or pork.
3. Choose high-quality meats that are raised without antibiotics or growth hormones.
4. Choose grass-fed beef whenever possible, and limit your beef consumption to help your heart and help the planet.
5. Eat seafood that is determined to be "Eco-Best." See www.edf.org/page.cfm?tagID=1521.

YOUR MOM WAS SO RIGHT

Win and Lose with Fruits and Vegetables

> *What did the carrot say to the wheat?*
> *"'Lettuce' rest, I'm feeling 'beet.'"*
> — Shel Silverstein

F THEY AREN'T ALREADY, make veggies your new best friends. Train yourself to be excited when you see an opportunity to eat them. They are critical for good health and for eliminating the fat on your body forever without your having to think or obsess about being fat again. Eat them raw. Sauté them in olive oil. Add them to soups. Make stir-fries with them. Pile salads high with them. Add them to your eggs. Throw them in your pasta sauces and enchiladas. Don't skimp. Load up on your veggies. Eat them all day long if you want. There are entire books on just the benefits of vegetables. They keep your body running and keep you feeling full and satisfied so you don't eat foods that you shouldn't, foods that are not on the List.

Veggies won't make you fat unless you cover them with

cheese, submerge them in fattening dips, or drown them in creamy sauces. This should be painfully obvious, but when you see spinach or artichoke dip on a menu or at a dinner party and think that might be a great way to get some necessary veggies in your diet — think again! The enormous fat content far outweighs any nutritional benefit you'd get from the spinach or artichoke hearts.

So far, I haven't found one vegetable I couldn't throw in a pan, lightly douse with canola, walnut, or olive oil, sprinkle with sea salt and freshly ground pepper, and broil in the oven until slightly browned and crispy that hasn't tasted amazing. My favorites are brussels sprouts, asparagus, green beans, sweet potato "fries," broccoli, cauliflower, and carrots. The prep time is about sixty seconds, so it's definitely worth checking out. One word of completely unsubstantiated advice concerning brussels sprouts: you can overdose on them, and it's not pretty. Let's just say if you can eat twenty or so medium-size brussels sprouts in one sitting and keep them all down, you're a lot tougher than I am. My mom had a similar experience. Strangely, hurling large amounts of brussels sprouts hasn't stopped me from continuing to eat them. Good thing!

I prefer fruits and vegetables purchased from natural grocery stores, farmers' markets, and local farms, but I also keep plenty of frozen and even canned veggies on hand. According to food expert Joy Bauer, author of *The Complete Idiot's Guide to Total Nutrition*, frozen and canned vegetables are just as good as or better than what you may find in your average produce section because they are packaged at peak freshness. Some so-called fresh produce has traveled quite a distance before it arrives at your grocery store. Bauer reminds us to read labels carefully to make sure salt, sugar, or fat hasn't been added for flavor or preservation reasons. She also says cooking vegetables doesn't necessarily remove the nutrients. Overboiling vegetables can cause this, but steaming and roasting vegetables help to retain flavor and nutritional value.

I could go on and on about how certain fruits can prevent the common cold or this vegetable improves your vision and that vegetable lowers your blood pressure, but that information is readily available, and I don't pay much attention to it anyway. Instead, I eat a variety of colorful fruits and vegetables throughout the day and make sure to eat five to nine servings daily. That seems like a lot, but according to 5aday.org, a serving size is:

- One medium-size piece of fruit
- ½ cup raw, cooked, frozen, or canned fruits or vegetables
- ¾ cup (6 oz.) 100 percent fruit or vegetable juice
- ½ cup cooked, canned, or frozen legumes (beans and peas)
- 1 cup raw, leafy vegetables

Colorful foods like sweet potatoes, beets, tomatoes, and blueberries (and even raw honey, molasses, and cinnamon) are considered *superfoods*. A superfood is a food rich in phytochemicals, which are special chemicals derived from certain plants that are said to prevent a multitude of diseases, cancers, and other ailments. Basically, they *phyte* all the bad stuff. Sounds like a *super* idea to me.

It gets even better. There's really no end to all the good stuff organic fruits and vegetables do for your body. Many plant-based food items (including whole grains) contain antioxidants. Unscientifically speaking, the body has a bazillion cells that are in a constant state of threat. One of those threats is free radicals. They can do some serious damage to cell membranes, can mutate the code in a single strand of DNA, and can trap bad cholesterol inside your artery walls. They are thought to contribute to cancer, atherosclerosis, and other chronic and life-threatening conditions. There is no escaping free radicals. They are generated as a natural consequence of food being converted into energy, and some are in the food we eat and the air we breathe. Antioxidants are our defense against these suckers, and they also slow down the aging process. I *really* like that last part. The Harvard School of Public Health website says there's no concrete evidence that antioxidant supplements will do much to neutralize free radicals; instead, antioxidants should come from the food we eat. There are many types of antioxidants and many foods that contain them. It gets a bit complicated, with polyphenols, flavonoids, carotenoids, androids, R2-D2, C-3PO, and the rest of the do-gooders, but suffice it to say, colorful fruits and vegetables, as well as whole grains, are a terrific source of these important antioxidants.

When I go grocery shopping, I start in the produce section, and by the time I'm ready to check out, at least half my cart is filled with assorted fruits and vegetables, and the rest is meat, dairy, grains, and other staples. I listen to my body (not literally) and see my doctor regularly to be sure I'm not lacking in any nutrients.

Fruit is usually an easy sell, but naked veggies are nature's biggest marvel. (Did I really just use the word *marvel*? I'm sticking with it.) Eat your veggies, just like your mom told you to. Of course, there are those who say they don't like veggies, and I think more men are guilty of this. Guess what, fellas? Just because some of you like to play video games, still think farting is funny, and watch *The Simpsons* and *Family Guy* doesn't mean you're actually twelve years old. Here's a news flash: YOUR TASTE BUDS CHANGE AS YOU AGE! I apologize for shouting, but you'd probably like a variety of vegetables by now, so give them a try. Pretty please?

ITEM #9: YOUR MOM WAS SO RIGHT

1. Eat a variety of colorful fruits and veggies every day.
2. Sauté veggies in heart-healthy oils like canola and olive oil.
3. Avoid eating fattening dips, sauces, and melted cheese with your vegetables.

GIMMICKS, SUPPLEMENTS, AND THE HYPE

THE FOOD INDUSTRY is constantly introducing products that promise new, incredible health benefits — sugar substitutes, energy drinks, cooking sprays, or fat-free versions of things I've been eating for years. I believe we should be eating food that was available long before any of us were even here, like eggs, milk, meat, nuts, fruits, vegetables — real food that fuels our bodies.

I also believe that eating a balanced diet consisting of a variety of foods, including plenty of fruits and vegetables, ensures that I'm getting all the nutrients I need for maximum health. However, I've been noticing that more and more doctors, as well as the Harvard School of Public Health, are recommending a daily multivitamin and that new studies show that getting the daily requirement through a supplement may help prevent heart disease, cancer, osteoporosis, and other chronic diseases. I'm not completely convinced.

I went to a natural grocery store recently to check out its vitamin and supplement section and found it incredibly overwhelming. It's going to take me a while to sort it all out before

I go filling my bathroom cabinet with a bunch of expensive bottles or even one that claims to do it all. In the end, I may stick to my belief that eating five to nine servings of assorted and colorful organic fruits and vegetables every day and eating a balanced diet does the trick perfectly. I'm skeptical, but a daily food-based multivitamin might be the way to go. I will make sure my multivitamin has "USP" on the label, which means it has passed purity and absorption tests and the vitamins won't just pass through my body without doing some good. Do what makes sense to you and your health care provider.

GOT FAT?

*Cholesterol, Good and Bad Fats,
and the Superstar Omega-3s*

> *When you die, if you get a choice between going
> to regular heaven or pie heaven, choose pie heaven.
> It might be a trick, but if not ... mmmmm, boy!*
> — Jack Handey

B EFORE YOU GET TO MR. HANDEY'S PIE HEAVEN, while you're still alive and kicking, there are good fats and bad fats. You need some fat, but it is important to understand why and to know the difference between good and bad fats. Bad fats are saturated fats and trans fats. Let's get to the big fat bottom of trans fats. Trans fats have other names, like partially or fully hydrogenated oils or trans fatty acids. Take a wild guess why there are multiple names for the same toxic substance. To confuse you. Don't be duped. Trans fats are fat substitutes that rob your body of the good fat that it actually needs to be optimally healthy. Oh, and they're poison — like arsenic. The definition of poison is "something that interferes with the metabolic processes of life by taking the place of a natural substance that performs a critical function." That's a mouthful, and one I sure didn't learn in college, but that's exactly what trans fats do. Your body cannot defend itself against them — it can't even digest them — so when you consume them, you are literally poisoning yourself, by choice. Slight amounts of trans fats occur naturally in foods like butter and other dairy products, but when they're added to hundreds of items like protein bars, frozen food, and baked goods, you need to be mindful of what the labels say. Fast food is another big culprit. Worrying about trans fats may someday be a thing of the past. New York, Philadelphia, and other cities have banned them in restaurants, and in 2008 California was the first state to do so.

At least for now, the issue of trans fats is still very present as well as overly confusing and full of tricky wording. While trans fats, or trans fatty acids, are critical to avoid, essential fatty acids, found in foods like fish, olives, nuts, and egg yolks, are critical to every metabolic function that occurs in your body. Your body is on a mission to get a sufficient amount of them. You will continue to feel hungry until you satisfy this bodily need. Since trans fats don't meet this need, they cause you to gain weight by forcing you to consume even more fat in order to get the essential fatty acids your body requires. Don't be bossed around by poison. That's not all. Trans fats also interfere with your body's ability to utilize the necessary fats that facilitate weight loss and heart health. So let's review how lousy trans fats are for you: They poison your body and create disease. They cause you to gain weight by telling your brain to go on a fat-seeking mission. And they interfere with all the great things that good fats do for you. Again, reading labels is an absolute must, and foods with hydrogenated oils, trans fatty acids, or trans fats are not on the List.

We've mentioned the perils of saturated fats found in beef and higher-fat dairy products. It's critical for your health and longevity to keep most saturated fats to a minimum. I say "most" because not all saturated fats are created equal. One exception to the saturated-fat rule may be coconut. According to Nina Planck, author of *Real Food: What to Eat and Why*, coconut flakes, milk, and oil contain lauric acid, an immune-boosting antiviral and antibacterial fatty acid that is also found in breast milk. Babies aren't the only ones who benefit from a strong and healthy immune system! In addition, a 2004 study says coconut oil keeps the important ratio between good and bad cholesterol in check (more on cholesterol in a minute). The study, conducted at the USDA's Diet and Human Performance Laboratory, found that "some foods that are rich in saturated fat contain protective, healthy nutrients as well. Chocolate, for instance, contains antioxidants and anti-platelet factors. Coconut also contains antioxidants. There is some evidence that these benefits may help outweigh the risks from the saturated fat. But most experts believe it is still not good to eat large amounts of these foods." And Dr. Oz reminds us that "all saturated fat speeds up aging," and "if you feast on foods rich in saturated fat you are much more likely to develop dementia." Being moderate and exercising common sense is the key. I love dark chocolate, and I strongly believe that it has many health-promoting attributes, but I wouldn't think of consuming an entire bar. I eat about one-tenth of a bar as my daily sweet treat.

The bad saturated fats are easy to spot because they are usually solid at room temperature — think cheese, butter, margarine, meat fat (lard), and chicken skin. Bad fats can clog your arteries and cause cardiovascular disease. The American Heart Association recommends that no more than 7 percent of your daily calories come from saturated fats. On a 1,500-calories-a-day plan, that's roughly 100 calories of saturated fats. Lightly butter two pieces of toast, and you've reached your limit. Two strips of bacon have roughly the same amount. A better idea is to skip the butter and the bacon, because small amounts of saturated fat exist in many of the healthy foods you eat, such as eggs, dark chocolate, chicken, and soy.

Generally speaking, good fats are monounsaturated and polyunsaturated fats, and they can lower the risk of disease. The folks at the Harvard School of Public Health say, "The key to a healthy diet is to substitute good fats for bad fats — and to avoid trans fats." They also say that while it is important to watch your cholesterol intake, it is more crucial to monitor the level of cholesterol in your bloodstream. The combination of fats you ingest, not the quantity of cholesterol you consume, makes the largest impact on your blood cholesterol. Cholesterol is a big-time factor in heart disease, which is the number one killer of both women and men in the United States today. It's important to get your numbers checked and gain control of your cholesterol.

ITEM #10: GOT FAT?

The deal with cholesterol can seem a bit complex, but there are really only three numbers to be mindful of: your LDL (low-density lipoproteins), HDL (high-density lipoproteins), and triglycerides. (If you don't care about the *why* and want to skip to the *how*, feel free to jump to the next paragraph.) Too much LDL can create plaque, which can narrow your arteries and restrict blood flow. The Harvard School of Public Health says, "When plaque breaks apart, it can cause a heart attack or stroke. Because of this, LDL cholesterol is often referred to as bad, or harmful, cholesterol." On the contrary, they say, "High-density lipoproteins (HDL) scavenge cholesterol from the bloodstream, from LDL, and from artery walls and ferry it back to the liver for disposal. Think of HDL as the garbage trucks of the bloodstream. HDL cholesterol is often referred to as good, or protective, cholesterol. Triglycerides make up most of the fat that you eat and that travels through the bloodstream. As the body's main vehicle for transporting fats to cells, triglycerides are important for good health. But as is the case for so many things, an excess of triglycerides can be unhealthy." Eating one cup of berries every day might boost your HDL levels, lower your blood pressure, and make you smile. The *American Journal of Clinical Nutrition* reported that study patients who did so had an increase in this good cholesterol by a little over 5 percent. Every little bit helps.

To maintain good cholesterol levels, go for *un*saturated fats. Unsaturated, good fats satiate you and make you feel full and satisfied because they slow down the absorption of food in your stomach. Have you figured out by now that slow digestion and absorption of food is a critical component to losing the extra weight and maintaining your ideal body weight? Examples of foods containing monounsaturated, good fats are canola, peanut, and olive oils, avocados, almonds, hazelnuts, pecans, pumpkin seeds, and sesame seeds. Polyunsaturated fats — including the superstars of the good-fat category, omega-3 fatty acids — benefit your heart and your immune system and are necessary for optimum metabolism. They increase your metabolic rate and ability to burn fat, which can result in weight loss. They also transport fat-soluble vitamins to your organs, cushion and protect your organs, and are necessary for optimal brain health. You can find these essential fatty acids in a variety of foods, such as ground flax seeds, walnuts, salmon, tuna, mackerel, and sardines, as well as in flax, soybean, sunflower, corn, walnut, and hempseed oil. Sauté your vegetables in one of these oils so you're sure to get some necessary good fat every day.

Please don't be tempted to use cooking sprays. As I previously mentioned, many contain alcohol, chemical propellants, or additives, and the can ends up in a landfill. Plus, you are robbing yourself of the opportunity to get the good fat you need from oils that are on the List. To use oil sparingly, invest in a manual pump designed to spray oil onto foods or into your pan before sautéing. Most kitchen stores sell them for ten or twenty dollars. A less expensive option that I use regularly is a small brush designed to lightly coat foods with oil or sauce.

ITEM #10: GOT FAT?

ITEM #10: *GOT FAT?*

1. Avoid most saturated fats and all trans fats.
2. Eat monounsaturated and polyunsaturated good fats, like almonds, avocados, and sesame seeds, and foods containing important omega-3 fatty acids, such as salmon, tuna, olive oil, and walnuts.
3. Avoid cooking sprays. Use a manual spray pump or small brush to lightly coat foods with good oils like olive, walnut, canola, and flax.

139

LEAN AND GREEN

Getting Lean Means Better Planetary Health

*We can't solve problems by using the same kind
of thinking we used when we created them.*
— Albert Einstein

EATING FOODS ON THE LIST not only transforms your body
and makes you healthier; it also helps transform the Earth
and makes our planet healthier. The foods you choose can
reduce the impact you make on Mother Earth. You are requiring less energy from the planet when you eat food that is minimally processed. When you choose whole grains, the planet's
energy and resources aren't expended taking apart the grain and
processing, refining, and bleaching it. Those whole grains
you're eating *are* eventually processed or broken down, though.
Guess where that energy comes from? *You!* So not only are you
saving Earth's precious resources and the energy required to
process whole grains into white foods; your body is using its
energy to break down those whole grains instead. That's good

news for you. When your body uses more energy, you become less fat. With white foods, all the good stuff, like the nutrients and the fiber, are thrown away and end up as waste. By eating whole grains, you are conserving the planet's energy, becoming less fat, and being less wasteful. Another way to cut back on waste is to choose real, whole, raw foods like fruits, vegetables, nuts, and whole grains, which use less packaging than processed and prepared foods.

Eating foods on the List makes you lean *and* green. While you're losing fat, becoming a smaller you, consuming only what you need, purchasing fewer packaged foods, and eating fewer refined foods, you are making a smaller impact on the Earth. Less impact is good. The name for this in green terminology is "reducing your carbon footprint." A carbon footprint is the amount of greenhouse gas emissions a person produces through his or her activities. Believe me, I'm not an alarmist. In my supersmart, serious-minded, know-it-all family, I'm the superficial, lighthearted one, and I tend to remain overly optimistic and hopeful in the face of challenge and difficulty. Plus, I get bored easily and find it excruciatingly painful to listen to their long, drawn-out lectures about the state of the planet. But when it comes to decreasing carbon dioxide and other emissions of greenhouse gases, you and I can't be that relaxed. That's what we've been doing, and it's not working. We are rapidly plunging into a major crisis, and every single one of us needs to step up and make drastic changes or we're not going to have to worry about Social Security, college savings, getting Alzheimer's, or looking cute in our designer denim because we cooked our planet . . . or at least cranked up the heat too high.

There are countless ways to reduce your carbon footprint in an effort to curb global warming, such as flying less, walking or biking to work, adjusting your thermostat, using energy-efficient lightbulbs, living in a smaller home, installing solar panels, moving to an urban area, getting rid of your lawn and planting a drought-tolerant native garden instead (or at least not watering your lawn, and ditching your gas-powered lawn mower for a manual version), buying food from local sources, and reducing the number of new things you use and purchase, like cars, grocery store bags, furniture, and even (*cringe*) designer jeans. By adopting some of these practices, you'll not only be making a difference and doing your part; you'll significantly stretch your dollar.

My love of fashion would create a serious problem with my bank account and credit card balances if I didn't habitually shop vintage and resale. Many resale boutiques sell new-to-you shoes and clothing for men and women and specialize in current, red-hot styles. I've found countless pairs of two-hundred-dollar jeans for thirty bucks. I'm also nuts about vintage clothing (and shoes, furniture, purses, scarves, and jewelry) and not above shopping at thrift stores, either. Don't think of it as used; think of it as recycling and doing your part to reduce waste as you're reducing your waist! Thanks to websites like Craigslist.org and Freecycle.org, new-to-you stuff is just a mouse-click away. Even better, five hundred tons of used items are not being thrown into landfills every day, resulting in enough stuff to fill a stack of garbage trucks five times the height of Mt. Everest each year.

Doing something as simple as bringing your own bags to the grocery store instead of taking new ones has a far-reaching impact. The *Wall Street Journal* reported that the United States consumes 100 billion plastic shopping bags every year. It takes roughly 12 million barrels of oil to make that many plastic bags. In addition to not consuming or buying so many brand-spanking-new things, we need to stop thinking about global warming and climate change as a political issue or even a national issue; it's a *global* issue, and we need to set our differences, finger pointing, and excuse making aside and scrape the yucky brown stuff off the fan together. At this late stage, who gives a crap (absolutely my last pun) how we got here? Let's open our eyes and see things as they are and make sweeping, radical changes so the Earth doesn't become uninhabitable. If some of the world's smartest scientists are wrong and global warming and climate change are just a natural and inevitable cycle, then *great!* Regardless, shouldn't we do everything in our power to slow down this process? If we don't, the price we will pay will be positively earth-shattering. (Time for the punitentiary?)

ITEM #11: LEAN AND GREEN

1. Choose whole foods such as whole grains, nuts, seeds, fruits, and vegetables that use *your* energy — instead of

ITEM #11: LEAN AND GREEN

Earth's energy and resources — for processing and require less packaging.

2. Significantly reduce your carbon footprint: fly less, walk or bike to work, live in a small home, move to an urban area, buy food only from local sources, and reuse items instead of constantly buying new things.

3. Bring bags with you whenever you go shopping.

CHEATING

MY SISTER ISN'T READY TO DEVIATE from her new habits, not even on isolated occasions. She will at some point — when she trusts herself enough to realize that a few dietary indiscretions every so often won't hurt her much in the long or short run. She was overweight her entire life (which I'm sure she appreciates my reminding you) and wants to make sure she's never fat again. She's afraid of what will happen if she steps over the line. Truth is . . . very little will happen. I cheat occasionally. I don't eat an entire chocolate cake or anything — they're little, tiny cheats.

On that road trip through Texas, when I stopped at Dairy Queen, what I didn't mention is that I had a kiddy-size vanilla ice cream cone. Not on the List, right? So it added a hundred empty calories to my day that may have been stored as fat. So the following day I was a little more vigilant — about a hundred calories or so more vigilant. No extremes here. On those days after cheating, maybe I'll skip that square of dark chocolate or eat half of a sandwich at lunchtime instead of the whole thing.

I know my body, and I trust myself. I've had many other indis-cretions over the years; I'm a serial cheater, indulging in a sug-ary cocktail at a New Year's Eve party or a slice of pepperoni pizza on white crust at a kid's birthday party. And you better believe I'll be eating a piece of cake at my children's weddings (I just hope one of them picks carrot cake with cream cheese frosting). When I cheat, I enjoy it completely and don't have the slightest bit of guilt. I balance it out over the following day or several days, and all is forgiven. The secret is, I don't make it a habit. Aha!

ITEM #12

TEN A.M. AND THREE P.M.

Snacking: Midmorning and Midafternoon, but Never Midnight

We must eat to live and not live to eat.
— *Molière*

I'M A HUGE FAN OF SNACKING. I think you should eat when you're hungry. If it has been three hours since lunch and you feel a little hungry, eat something! Eating keeps your metabolism revving at maximum speed. Plus, eating a healthy snack prevents you from overeating at the next meal. Rather than tell you what's not on the List, I've made some suggestions of snacks that are — it's a mini-list, not *the* List.

Snacks are best eaten at midmorning or midafternoon; never eat them at midnight. Actually, it is rare for me to eat anything after dinner. I also make sure to eat dinner a few hours before I go to bed so my body has a chance to burn off some of my meal. Eating right before bed is a superb way to ensure that your body stores your dinner or snack as fat. If I do any postdinner snacking, I go for a bowl of blueberries or strawberries. I prefer snacks that require zero prep time. Fruit makes an ideal choice. Each week, I restock the giant fruit bowl that I keep on the kitchen island. It is the first thing I notice when I enter the kitchen and is a beautiful reminder to load up on vitamins, minerals, and important enzymes.

What happens when we feel a tiny hunger pang and find ourselves staring at the kitchen pantry or standing in front of the fridge? We think we're hungry, right? I find that a good seven out of ten times, I actually just need a glass of water. The other 30 percent of the time, I don't need much — just a tiny refuel. A whole wheat cracker with a teaspoon of peanut butter or a few walnuts and a small piece of dark chocolate do the trick. Snacks don't need to be big.

When you're snacking — or anytime — I caution you to avoid packaged foods and learn to carefully read labels. Packaged foods often contain trans fats, high fructose corn syrup, or far too much sodium. Some sodium is necessary for your body, but when you consume too much, your kidneys can't filter it effectively, which causes it to accumulate in your blood and actually makes your blood volume increase. This increase in blood overworks your heart and puts extra pressure on your arteries. Remember the last time you were at a party and ate half the cheese, olive, smoked salmon, and salami plate? Do you recall how your clothes felt the next day? Like they were cutting off your circulation? That delightful bloated sensation is likely from excessive sodium intake.

ITEM #12: TEN A.M. AND THREE P.M.

If you eat a ton of "diet" or packaged foods, you're probably overdosing on sodium. MayoClinic.com says that 77 percent of our sodium intake comes from packaged or prepared foods. Make a serious and conscious effort to cut down on packaged foods. Those so-called diet and fat-free foods like Lean Cuisine and Healthy Choice? Have you ever read the list of ingredients on one of those frozen meals? Lean Cuisine's Baked Chicken, for example, contains both HFCS and partially hydrogenated soybean and/or cottonseed oils as well as a very long list of ingredients that didn't exist when your grandmother was a child. Oh, and it also contains 27 percent of your recommended daily allowance of sodium. And please don't get me started on those ridiculous 100-calorie snack packs. I'm not a fan because I eat real food. It goes beyond the fake ingredients, heavy packaging, and high sodium content, though. They don't fill you up! Real foods with fiber and bulk are far more satiating. If you buy packaged food like butter, peanut butter, soup, or tuna, choose the low- or no-sodium version. You can always add a little salt for flavor if you feel the need.

Do yourself a monstrous favor, and buy sea salt instead of iodized table salt. Iodized table salt typically contains aluminum and bleach, whereas sea salt is just evaporated seawater. Sea salt is also more flavorful, so when I add it to recipes like baked goods, sauces, or tuna salad, I tend to use less than the recipes call for. If you're worried about missing out on necessary iodine, you can get it from other foods, such as fish, shellfish, strawberries, yogurt, milk, and eggs. For optimum purity and health, try Himalayan pink salt. This hand-mined salt, harvested from ancient sea salt deposits, comes from the foothills of the Himalayan mountains and is rich in minerals like iron, calcium, magnesium, and potassium. You can find it at gourmet grocery stores.

If you don't get hungry between meals and seem to manage well on eating three squares, by all means, do what works for you. If you're like me and need a snack to keep your energy going, here are some of my faves:

- Small serving of edamame (salted green soybeans)
- Tossed garden salad
- Piece of fruit or mixed-fruit salad
- Light string cheese
- Half cup of 100 percent–fruit applesauce
- Hard-boiled, scrambled, or poached egg on whole grain toast
- Scoop of tuna salad or egg salad in whole wheat pita
- Cup of soup — broth-, tomato-, or legume-based
- Handful of raisins
- Whole grain toast with pure peanut butter and low- or no-sugar jam
- Small bowl of whole grain cereal
- Small bowl of oatmeal
- Sautéed or steamed veggies with half cup of brown rice or quinoa
- Four slices of turkey rolled up with avocado

ITEM #12: TEN A.M. AND THREE P.M.

- Half of a tuna, turkey, or chicken sandwich on whole wheat bread
- Handful of whole wheat crackers with egg-white salad
- Popcorn cooked in olive oil and a small amount of sea salt
- Carrot sticks dipped in one tablespoon of organic ranch dressing
- Celery dipped in one tablespoon of pure peanut or almond butter
- Small handful of almonds, peanuts, or walnuts
- Scoop of hummus in whole wheat pita
- Whole grain tortilla with grilled chicken and one tablespoon shredded mozzarella cheese (part-skim)
- Half cup of cottage cheese with fruit
- Nonfat plain yogurt with berries and honey, agave nectar, or raw brown sugar
- One small square of dark chocolate

Did you know that eating dark chocolate is good for you? It's a potent antioxidant. Remember the good deeds that antioxidants do for your body? They gobble up free radicals (destructive molecules), which are implicated in heart disease and cancer. To me, there is nothing better than a small square of dark chocolate in the midafternoon. Not all dark chocolate is the same, though. The higher the cocoa content, the better for you. I eat only 70 percent or higher. My favorite is 85 percent, which does take some getting used to, but I swear it makes me feel instantly happier.

SNACKING AND KIDS

I realize that, from the Introduction and the story I'm about to share with you, it may seem like I'm picking on soccer moms. On the contrary, I used to be a soccer mom — a really annoying one. The kind that complained about all the sugary halftime and postgame snacks the kids were eating, to the point that I was asked to step down as the volunteer team-parent-slash-manager of my son's kindergarten soccer team. I politely refused. I felt the team needed me. By the time my son played classic soccer in sixth grade, I was having coaches fired. It was actually just one coach. He told the boys they were "playing like girls" and that his mom could run faster than they could. Before I wrote an angry letter to the club's director, I reminded the coach that his girl's team had just won the state championship and that I would personally like to challenge him to a fifty-yard dash. I am so grateful he declined. That was the end of Coach "Manly Man" as well as Kami "The Interferer" as a soccer mom, but it served as my training in how to dress one, which proved quite useful later on.

My point? I get pretty fired up about kids and sports, particularly all the crap "well-meaning" parents are feeding kids during and after games and practices. I don't get it. The only thing kids need when they're playing sports is water — and maybe a few orange slices at halftime. I don't want my child to drink a juice box (with no real juice in it) and eat a chewy chocolate chip granola bar that contains over forty ingredients, including high fructose corn syrup and trans fat, at 10:30 in the morning in the middle of his soccer game. Or ever. By 10:30, he's already had breakfast and doesn't need the spike in his sugar levels that consequently makes him a lousy second-half player and a cranky, hyper, and insufferable brat on the car ride home. If I don't allow him to indulge, I'm the mean, strict parent who gets uptight about something as seemingly harmless as a granola bar, or a Krispy Kreme doughnut, or "fruit" shaped like Teenage Mutant Ninja Turtles. I see some of these same parents buying expensive, healthy, gourmet dog food for Tiger and then feeding their children a bunch of fake, fattening, processed food. Don't even get me started on the end-of-the-season party with pizza, cake, and candy! In my perfectly healthy world, the end of the season would be celebrated with a tasty barbecue of grilled chicken, corn on the cob, fruit salad, and whole wheat strawberry shortcake.

I'll get off my soapbox, but kids are innocent victims and don't have much say in what they eat. That's the beauty. We parents get to decide. As we make better decisions for ourselves, let's let the kids in on it. I'm not saying control everything they put in their mouths. That would be impossible. Just make sure that common sense is exercised most of the time — like when they're playing sports. On their birthdays, break out the chocolate cupcakes and vanilla ice cream. If you really want to give them a treat, make the cupcakes yourself with real, organic, wholesome ingredients.

ITEM #12: TEN A.M. AND THREE P.M.

1. Eat a small, healthy snack when you're hungry.
2. Snack at midmorning and midafternoon but never at midnight.
3. If you snack after dinner, make sure it is minimal and eaten a few hours before you go to bed.
4. Eat real food, not fake, "lite," "diet," "fat-free" packaged foods, which can be high in sodium and full of nasty fillers.
5. Use unbleached, mineral-rich sea salt instead of iodized table salt.

I LIKE THE WAY YOU MOVE

Customize the Way You Exercise

> *So ask your doctor if getting*
> *off your ass is right for you!*
> *— Bill Maher*

MOVING AROUND IS IMPORTANT. I believe *how* you move around is less important. Physical activity can be vigorous sweeping, yoga classes, a daily walk or visit to the gym, training for a triathlon, or my personal favorite, dancing around the house to Madonna, Duran Duran, or Elton John's "Crocodile Rock." I wish I didn't, but I detest the gym and rarely stick with any exercise routine for more than six months to a year. But I'm extremely active and my job is pretty labor-intensive. I move quickly, walk fast, and take the stairs as often as possible. I once gave up my car and biked everywhere for six months straight, but that was because I was too cheap to help my daughter buy a car, so I gave her mine. (The one time I tried to buy her some wheels, I answered an ad for a used car and my daughter and I met some creepy guy in a deserted parking lot. We were pretty convinced the guy had recently stolen the car. She thought so because he was wearing a black leather jacket, had greasy hair, and was smoking a cigarette. I thought so because someone's laptop and a pair of high heels were lying in the backseat. The owner was probably in the trunk. We literally sprinted back to our car before he had a chance to kill us and sell our organs on eBay.) Find some way to be active: garden, take a Pilates class, chase your children or grandchildren around the park, go swimming or jogging, work out with weights, take a ballet or tap class, or go to Jazzercise — but get a move on!

Maybe you think Jazzercise is corny, but it is a killer workout! Plus, corny is the new cool! The three times in my life that I've been in seriously amazing shape were when I was taking Jazzercise classes three or four days a week. An hour-long class goes by quickly because you're dancing to poppy tunes and working out with weights, bands, and exercise balls. It's not at all an intimidating atmosphere, and the folks who run it are always ridiculously friendly and welcoming. The guy who operates the center near my house is some kind of Jazzercise celebrity and travels all over the world for the company. I took a class while traveling in Canada, and the students literally screamed like rock star groupies when I told them who my hometown Jazzercise instructor was. They kept asking me to demonstrate how my guru did certain routines and *oooh*ed and *ahh*ed when I showed them. I must say, I kind of liked the attention.

Whatever you choose, regular physical exercise is hugely beneficial to your overall health and significantly contributes to weight loss and maintenance. Activities that involve light weights or stretching are especially helpful. Weight-bearing exercises are essential for optimum bone health and can help prevent bone loss or osteoporosis.

Making exercise part of a regular routine is tough for many people. A doctor and dear friend of mine who works full-time in her busy dermatology practice and has five kids decided one day that even though she had a million legitimate excuses to not find the time to exercise, making excuses was no longer going to be an option. She had no desire to waste precious time and energy driving to and from a gym, so she bought some light weights, a twenty-minute Pilates DVD, and a rowing machine. She committed to getting up an hour earlier each day. My friend loves to read, so to help pass the time, she listens to audiobooks on her iPod during her workout. She says this has become a real motivator because she wakes up looking forward to hearing more of her book. She also says it's not the fat-burning or health aspect of her workout that keeps her from hitting the snooze button. She just gets up, mindlessly throws on some workout wear, and hits Play on her iPod.

As you lose the fat, you will notice that you have more spring in your step; you'll feel bouncier and lighter because you *are* lighter. Before long, taking the stairs and walking from here to there won't tire you as quickly. By substituting twenty minutes a day of walking for driving, the average person could lose as much as seven pounds in a year without changing any other habits. I have to shop a great deal for work. I purposefully park my car as far away from my target destination (which, coincidentally, is often Target) as possible, ensuring that I'll have an opportunity to get my heart rate up a bit. If I'm schlepping bags on the way back to my car, I get even more of a boost.

Being good to your body and moving more can also help you make less impact on the planet. Weather permitting, biking or walking to work or the neighbor's house or the grocery store burns calories without requiring your car to burn through more fuel. If you can, take mass transit. I live six blocks from Portland's light rail system, called MAX. That's twelve blocks round-trip of walking for me, and I'm not blowing through any nonrenewable energy sources. I save a little money, and at the same time, my legs get shapelier and leaner (too bad no one will ever see them — they are so white I'd probably cause mass blindness if I wore a pair of shorts). Do what you can to move more. Every day. It all adds up to better health, increased longevity, weight loss and maintenance, and getting into that dream pair of jeans!

ITEM #13: I LIKE THE WAY YOU MOVE

1. Move more every day.
2. Take the stairs whenever possible.
3. Discover the joy of daily stretching and using light weights to maintain healthy bones.
4. Find activities that you enjoy, and mix it up.
5. Park your car far away from your destinations.
6. Walk to nearby stores, restaurants, or neighbors' houses.

EATS WELL WITH OTHERS

*Your Friends, Family,
and Favorite Food Enablers*

> *Never compromise yourself.
> You are all you've got.*
> — Betty Ford

I'M A SINGLE MOM. I have a nineteen-year-old daughter and a seventeen-year-old son. (Dad is the boyfriend I mentioned at the beginning of the book. We got married eight weeks after college graduation and discovered after seven years of marriage that the only thing we had in common outside of gaining weight in college and our deep and unwavering love for the most adorable kids ever was nothing actually.) When the kids were young, sometimes I made two different dinners, one for them and one for me. Occasionally, I let my kids eat potatoes, white pasta, white buns on their hamburgers, and even brownies with vanilla ice cream.

I allowed this for several reasons. First off, we all remember those kids from our own childhoods (or maybe you were one of them) who weren't allowed to eat certain things, like sweets or processed foods. What did those kids eat when they came to your house, and what did they purchase at the neighborhood grocery store? Bingo! All the forbidden foods! Since neither of my kids has a weight problem, I gave them a taste of everything so they wouldn't let curiosity and human nature get the best of them.

Second, I know from personal experience that we stray from what our parents taught us and showed us, but only temporarily if their lessons start to make sense to us as adults. My kids know what's on the List as well as I do and also know why things are on the List. My daughter rolled her eyes at me and made a nasty face when I asked her to read the manuscript for this book and give me her opinion. I guess she's heard my preaching for so long that she's not the least bit interested in a lengthy recap. Eighty percent of the time, my daughter chooses foods that are on the List. The rest of the time, she eats like a typical American teenager — like crap. She knows her body has the ability to increase in size. She's put it to the test; by only a few measly pounds, but she knows. Her jeans tell her, just as ours tell you and me. Hers are just way more expensive and completely shredded on the bottom from not having been hemmed properly and being worn with flip-flops.

My son, on the other hand, is getting away with bacon-double-cheeseburger murder. He's got a raging metabolism and eats like crap because he can — or he thinks he can. It won't last forever. No names here, but plenty of men in our family are fighting the ever-expanding spare tire around the old midsection. He'll know what to do when the time comes, and his mother can't wait! He's been half-listening to me his entire life, so he's armed with firsthand knowledge of the List, and I have every reason to believe that one day he'll swear by it.

My point being, your dinner plate may look slightly different from your children's, your spouse's, your significant other's, or your roommate's. You may even get hassled a bit or questioned by your loved ones. They'll eventually get used to it, and you'll get used to the extra effort it takes, which is a minor adjustment, really. They're having fried chicken? Remove the skin or outer coating, or even better, grill or bake yours. They're eating spaghetti with white noodles? Make a small pot of whole wheat spaghetti noodles for yourself. Skip the baked potato on steak night and have an extra helping of vegetable or salad instead. Have a bowl of blueberries while they're eating ice cream for dessert. Fruit sorbet you make yourself with fresh fruit, ice, and a small amount of fruit juice works too. Throw a few chopped raw almonds on top for added protein and crunch. You get the idea, right?

Prepare yourself for comments and concerns from family and friends (aka food enablers) about how you're "missing out" and "limiting yourself." Just remember, you are retraining yourself and developing habits to get rid of that excess fat you've been carrying around. Some people close to you will be curious. Some will be jealous. Some will criticize your methods and try to undermine your progress and newly developed habits. Some may try to guilt you into eating something you shouldn't by saying it's your favorite and they made it (or bought it) especially for you. Be gracious, and politely but firmly decline. Your best defense is not to be defensive. Be indifferent. Stay strong and chalk it up to human nature. Indifference is a powerful tool. Do what dogs do: silently tilt your head with a semipuzzled but trusting look, and go back to what you were doing.

You have control over your own mind and the choices you make and the habits you choose to develop. You also have the ability to change how you react when people question, criticize, or try to undermine you. Don't bother defending or explaining your choices if you don't want to. You have a right to them and you are not forcing them (literally or figuratively) down anyone else's throat. Be indifferent. When you're indifferent and not taking the bait, before long your friends, family, and co-workers will get bored, let it go, and move on. They'll see your energy level increase and your waistline decrease, and they'll stop questioning, commenting, and criticizing. Or they'll just lose interest. Trust yourself. Trust what your body is telling you. Trust your doctor to determine if your choices are creating a healthier body for you. You are strong and powerful and have control over your own mind and the choices and decisions you make. How amazing is that?

ITEM #14: EATS WELL WITH OTHERS

1. Unless everyone is on board, when dining at home with others, make slight modifications to your meal to make it List-approved.
2. Be indifferent when others express criticism or curiosity about your new choices and habits.
3. Trust yourself and your doctor to determine if your new choices and habits are creating a healthier you.

ITEM #15

COUNT ME IN!

Calories, Portions, and Proportion

*Reality is the murder of a beautiful theory
by a gang of ugly facts.*
— Robert Glass

NOT EVERYONE WILL NEED to pay strict attention to calories in order to succeed at losing weight and maintaining their ideal, healthy weight. If everything you put in your body has ' nutritional value, you make sure to eat a balanced diet, you don't eat beyond feeling full, and you're attentive to what your specific body needs in terms of portions, you can probably skip to the next chapter. I'm not one of those people. My friends and family joke that I'm part cow because I seem to have four stomachs. I have to be mindful of calories and portions because I rarely get full. I've tried the eating-very-slowly trick, which gives your meal time to send the "I'm full — stop eating now" signal to your brain before you eat the whole enchilada. That strategy works amazingly well for most people but, alas, not for me. I don't believe in being obsessive about counting calories, but for me, it matters.

At some point, usually every day, in my head I tally up where I am. I know what my body requires. I shoot for 1,500 calories a day but land anywhere from 1,300–1,800 depending on the day's events. I typically consume more calories on the weekends than I do on weekdays, and I consume less when eating at home versus eating out. I came up with my daily goal by trial and error, but you can also figure out your approximate basal metabolic rate (BMR) by using the Harris-Benedict formula, which has been around for almost ninety years. When you combine that with the amount of physical activity you engage in, you can get a pretty realistic idea of how many daily calories to aim for.

Either enter a few bits of information into the convenient BMR calculator at www.walking.about.com/cs/calories/1/blcalcalc.htm or (less fun) figure it out yourself:

WOMEN: BMR = 655 + (4.35 × weight in pounds) + (4.7 × height in inches) − (4.7 × age in years)

MEN: BMR = 66 + (6.23 × weight in pounds) + (12.7 × height in inches) − (6.8 × age in years)

Once you've arrived at that shocking figure, you get to bump it up a notch based on your level of physical activity, using the following formula:

ITEM #15: COUNT ME IN!

SEDENTARY $=$ BMR $\times$ 1.2 (little or no exercise, desk job)

LIGHTLY ACTIVE $=$ BMR $\times$ 1.375 (light exercise/ sports 1–3 days per week)

MODERATELY ACTIVE $=$ BMR $\times$ 1.55 (moderate exercise/ sports 3–5 days per week)

VERY ACTIVE $=$ BMR $\times$ 1.725 (hard exercise/sports 6–7 days per week)

EXTREMELY ACTIVE $=$ BMR $\times$ 1.9 (hard daily exercise/ sports and physical job or twice-daily marathon training)

These are just guidelines, and it's always a good idea to ask your doctor what he or she thinks would be a good daily goal for you while you're losing weight. According to the online BMR calculator, my BMR combined with a moderate level of activity computes to 1,940 calories, which means that to maintain my current weight, I can consume roughly that amount per day. This is higher than what I set as my target, but most people, including yours truly, underestimate the caloric content of the food they're eating. If you don't understand how calories add up, buy a book on calories or use a calorie counter on the Internet. The daily goal will be different for everyone, and men generally need more. It's all about portions and proportions.

My mom is barely five feet tall and weighs around a hundred pounds. She consumes fewer calories than I do. My mom used to be heavier and claimed it was due to being big-boned. Unlikely! When she was at her heaviest, she temporarily abandoned her good eating habits and dove into bags of potato chips and boxes of Wheat Thins, which she dipped in ranch dressing or onion dip that she made from powdered mixes. I think it was one of those years when she was extra pissed at my dad. These days, her portions at family meals are considerably smaller than mine are. Not only is she six inches shorter than I am and about twenty-five pounds lighter; she's twenty-four years older, which means her metabolism is likely slower. Proportionally, she needs to consume fewer calories than I do to maintain her ideal healthy body weight. I've got to believe she's eating enough food and calories, because she's a bundle of energy. My parents ski a few times a week during the winter (wearing adorable matching helmets) and Mom beats Dad down the mountain every run, and Dad is in pretty decent shape. (He made me write that.)

As you age, you will likely need to make slight adjustments to your diet to compensate for your changing and, sorry to say, slowing metabolism. I can't consume the number of calories I could ten years ago. It wouldn't hurt to keep a daily log of calories while you're losing weight and also when you're first learning to maintain your ideal weight. If you're eating only foods on the List and watching your portions (think deck of cards–size portions for meats and grains), you might assume that counting calories and keeping a daily food diary is a pointless exercise because the weight is coming off effortlessly, but it's also an important tool to ensure you're eating a balanced diet. I believe that whole grains, fruits, vegetables, dairy, protein, and good fats all need to be present in your diet for you to be optimally healthy.

The dermatologist friend I mentioned in Item #13 keeps a "health journal." Each day, she jots down what she eats and also keeps track of her physical activity, health concerns, and goals for the coming day. She updates her journal at night and also reviews the previous day's entry to see if she stuck to her plan. In other words, she checks in with herself for positive reinforcement and for a reminder to honor the commitments she's made to herself. Her journal is just for her and helps her maintain healthy habits.

One item my friend does not include in her health journal is how much she weighs. Like me, she uses her clothes to bear that news. Weighing yourself frequently, especially every day, is not such a great idea. Any number of factors — excessive water consumption or fluid retention, a plentiful meal, the time of day, the time of month, and so on — can create a weight fluctuation of up to five pounds. At the most, weigh yourself once a week or every ten days to gauge your progress, and let your jeans tell the rest of the story. Jumping on the scale each morning probably won't give you the answer you're looking for, and if it does, it'll say something different the following day. Rather than risk feeling defeated and obsessing over a daily weigh-in, make good choices, assess how your clothes are fitting you, and check your progress on the bathroom scale no more than three or four times a month. The big bottom line (get it?): calories do matter, but more important, eat real food consisting of low-GI carbs, lean proteins, good fats, and plenty of assorted and colorful fruits and vegetables; drink enough water to keep your body hydrated; get adequate exercise; and keep your portions in check.

ITEM #15: COUNT ME IN!

1. Ask your healthcare provider what a good daily goal is in terms of calories while you are losing and maintaining weight, or use the formula in this chapter.
2. Keep a daily log to ensure you're not consuming too many calories and that you're getting a balanced diet.
3. It's calories in, calories out, but what you eat matters. Eat real food consisting of low-GI, high-fiber carbs, lean proteins, good fats, and plenty of assorted and colorful fruits and vegetables, and drink enough water to keep your body hydrated.

Food for Thought

STAYING IN CONTROL

ONCE YOU ARE AT YOUR IDEAL HEALTHY WEIGHT, you may go through a stage in which you're afraid you're going to lose control. So you hold on tightly, maybe even become a little obsessive. I mentioned that my sister is currently going through something like this. It may even spill over into other areas of your life. This happened to me. After I lost the weight, graduated from college, got married, and settled into what I thought would be domestic bliss, I found myself obsessing over food because I feared I would get fat again. I needed a distraction, so I became fixated on my house being perfect at all times. In particular, I became obsessed with vacuuming my carpet. I was completely despondent if my carpet didn't have those vacuum cleaner trails going through it. So you know what I did? I installed wood floors. Actually, that was much later. I slowly learned to trust myself and eased up on the tension and energy I was expending to keep things under control — to keep the fat from coming back.

Take several deep, good-for-your-brain, cleansing breaths,

and remember, you have the power over your own mind. Be patient with yourself. When you find yourself being obsessive, focus on something else. Read a book or play with your kids. Go take a walk or see a movie. Realize that you may blow it occasionally. I make sure to stock my pantry and fridge only with foods on the List. I could overeat, but I couldn't eat gummy bears and ice cream because I never buy them.

Having said that, I realize that some of you live with other people and there are times when you'll buy items that are not intended for you and are not List-approved. What should you do? Select a special spot in the refrigerator, freezer, and pantry for items that are not on the List. I don't shop for him much anymore, but when my son brings his crap into our house, it goes in the designated spots. He's much taller than both me and his older sister, so he gets the top shelf in our pantry. I can barely reach it anyway, but that spot is off-limits to me, and I generally look at it with disdain. He'll figure out how to eat eventually, and meanwhile, I'm not the least bit tempted. Remember, it all starts with how you look at food — as fuel that makes your body lean, healthy, and full of energy.

In the back of the book (page 215) is a list to get you started on packing your pantry with healthy foods on the List. Remember to read labels carefully and look for foods that are certified organic, are fair trade if possible, and don't contain high fructose corn syrup or trans fats. If there's one in your area, shop at a farmers' market for the freshest fruits, vegetables, nuts, cheese, and coffee. To be less wasteful, bring your own bags to farmers' markets and grocery stores. Most grocery stores sell the perfect reusable grocery bag for around a buck. I have a bunch of them and use them for groceries but also for recycling and toting items to Goodwill. Don't be afraid to mix it up — store clerks won't give you the hairy eyeball if you bring a bright green Whole Foods bag to Trader Joe's — I do it all the time!

EATING AWAY FROM HOME

An Out-and-About Guide to Healthful Eating

> *While we may not be able to*
> *control all that happens to us,*
> *we can control what happens inside us.*
> — *Benjamin Franklin*

I EAT AT LEAST FIVE MEALS A WEEK away from home. Fast food aside, there is always something on a restaurant menu I can eat. I've become very skilled at reading menus and determining the best option. The problem is, I have this annoying habit of doing it for other people I'm dining with. I just get so excited about eating well. My kids used to have no idea how to peruse a menu because I always did it for them. I didn't order for them. I'd make suggestions, and they came to trust that I pretty much got it right every time. Plus, they knew if they put up too much of a fuss, they would have to endure a long, drawn-out lecture regarding choices and habits, and no kid wants that.

Before I break it down for you, I want to teach you a skill I use to maintain my good habits. I call it FPV, which sounds like an acronym for a newly discovered sexually transmitted disease, but it's short for Food Planning and Visualization, a helpful tool to use on your journey to fatlessness (yes, I have spellchecker). Now that so many restaurants have their menus online, FPV has become even easier. Think I'm off my rocker? I don't have a rocker just yet, so hear me out. The human mind is incredibly powerful. Successful people visualize their success before it happens. Take professional golfers. Did you know that the really great ones (or maybe all of them) plan out every stroke in their head before they ever swing the club? They visualize their swing, what the ball will do after it makes contact with the club, what path it will take, and exactly where it will land on the fairway or green.

In much the same way, I visualize what I'm going to eat. I plan it out beforehand. I do this several times a day. It has become habit for me. At night, I might review in my head what I ate that day and realize I went a little over the top, so I visualize what I will eat the next day. I make a plan. If I have a restaurant meal on my schedule, I picture items I know the place serves or check its website for a sneak preview of the menu. I believe planning and visualizing is an important exercise that can help you in your quest to lose and maintain weight. It may not be for everybody, but it works for me and has been an easy and effortless habit to develop.

Before I delve into all the great possibilities of healthy eating by restaurant type, I'll discuss some other places out in the world you may find yourself needing to fearlessly navigate.

ITEM #16: EATING AWAY FROM HOME

PARTIES AND POTLUCKS

I always eat a little something before I go to a dinner party. Since I have literally zero control over what will be served at the party, I supply my body with fuel beforehand so I don't completely lose it and eat an entire plate of cheese and crackers. The usual appetizers, hors d'oeuvres, and bowls of nuts are extra pounds in the making. Party hosts are apprehensive about serving starters that the average person doesn't eat or enjoy, so they usually offer fattening crowd-pleasers. I've been guilty of this as well, but I always provide a few tasty options that are on the List, like mini–tandoori chicken skewers, which are high in protein. One or two are the perfect pre-dinner snack. If there are no good choices, skip the starters altogether. Just sip on water, wine, or a vodka soda, and wait for the main course. If your hosts are serving a specialty cocktail and not serving wine until dinner, cheerfully decline and let them know that water is good for now.

For the main course, if it's something I absolutely don't eat, like white pasta with cream sauce, I've got a bit of a situation. Not a complete train wreck, but I will be relying heavily on the salad or vegetable. Plus, I don't want to make it blatantly obvious that I have a problem with the host's carefully planned and executed meal. So I do what four-year-olds do and pick at my food. I go on a mining expedition in search of protein and vegetables and move things around on my plate. And I hide the rest under a large lettuce leaf or two. I'm not kidding. If lean meat, beans, or lentils plus a vegetable or salad are being served, I'm over the moon. If

I'm allowed to fix my own plate, I load it with two-thirds veggies and one-third protein and have seconds of veggies if I'm still hungry. I want to be completely satiated when dessert arrives so I'm not the least bit tempted.

Dessert can be challenging if your host is putting one in front of each person at a sit-down dinner party. This just happened to me. Crème brûlée. It's much easier if you're asked first and you can respectfully decline by saying that dinner was so incredibly delicious that you don't have a smidgen of room left. A harder sell if you pulled the four-year-old trick and left most of the food on your plate. To deal with the crème brûlée, I picked at it and ate teeny-tiny bites until I had eaten the equivalent of one large bite, and sipped on decaf coffee. It was delicious, but not on the List. When my hostess asked if I wasn't a fan of her dessert, I simply said that I was too full, but I would sure love the recipe! (I can't lie to you. It wasn't actually crème brûlée, but if I say what the dessert really was, that person will know I'm talking about her [rhymes with *hairy beefsteak*], which in turn could cause some hurt feelings.) Obviously, if I know my hosts well and we are friends, they already know what a total pain in the ass I am. Therefore, I come clean and tell them their entire menu was an example of what *not* to eat and let them know I will be featuring them in my next book in a chapter titled "How to Fatten Up Your Friends in Just One Night!"

At birthday parties, office parties, and bridal or baby showers, there may not be any real food — just cake. Hopefully, you're well acquainted with the folks there, and you won't offend anyone by not being the first in line for a piece of cardboard-tasting grocery-store cake with imitation lemon filling and fake buttercream frosting (read: high fructose corn syrup and hydrogenated oils). Unless you're the guest of honor and it would clearly be rude to decline, you don't have to eat cake or drink punch to be the life of the party. You do have to sing "Happy Birthday," though. If you sing really loudly and obnoxiously like I do, maybe you won't be invited the next time, and problem solved!

Potlucks are a hideous mishmash of food and cookware, but they require very little thought in terms of making good choices because you get to bring something. I always assume there won't be any other items on the List, so I make my dish an entire meal, like meat and vegetable lasagna or enchiladas with chicken, quinoa, black beans, black olives, mushrooms, and onions. I bring my own lowfat sour cream to use sparingly on top. For some potlucks, you may be assigned a certain type of dish. When this happens and I arrive with something entirely different, I just smile and say "oops" and hope everyone else followed the rules. This backfired on me once, and we were stuck eating my chicken enchiladas for dessert. I offered to run out and get some fresh berries, but the hostess wanted to punish and embarrass me instead. She succeeded. Watch your portions at potlucks. Just because quite a few items appear to be on the List doesn't mean you need to try them all. I steer way clear of casseroles unless I made them or I know who made them, as they often include large amounts of cheese, cream, and unidentified ingredients and are best to avoid altogether.

BOWLING ALLEYS, STATE FAIRS, SPORTING EVENTS, AND THEME PARKS (PLUS ZOOS, MOVIE THEATERS, MALLS, AND MONSTER TRUCK RALLIES)

Eat before you go and bring your own snacks. With few exceptions, these venues serve garbage — expensive garbage that makes you fat. Great people watching, though.

AIRPORTS AND AIRPLANES

I'm sitting in the Dallas airport as I'm writing this, and I'm a little cranky, so I may go off a bit. I really need something to eat. I had to get up at four in the morning for my flight back home to Portland. My choices are beyond grim: Taco Bell, McDonald's, Starbucks, Dunkin' Donuts, Au Bon Pain, and the airport store. I head to Au Bon Pain for a made-to-order tuna or chicken sandwich on a nine-grain roll. I can see a small sign that clearly says NINE-GRAIN ROLLS, and a dozen or so rolls behind the sign in the pastry case. I place my order and the gal tells me that she's out of nine-grain rolls. I smile and point to the nine-grain rolls. She proceeds to tell me that those particular nine-grain rolls are for display only. I politely ask if it would be too much trouble to have my sandwich made on one of the display rolls. She says that is against company policy and she is already on probation for something else. Au Bon Pain in my ass.

The Starbucks only has sandwiches made on white bread,

so I head to the airport convenience store for a protein bar. Protein bars are at the bottom of the List. They are a last resort. They typically are high in protein and fiber but are also loaded with sugar and contain a bunch of mystery ingredients. Some have the dreaded high fructose corn syrup and some form of partially hydrogenated oil (trans fats). I found the least foul one of the bunch and bought a bag of raw almonds along with it. Eating a protein bar is better than not eating at all. It has now been twelve hours since I have had any food, and my metabolism is going downhill fast, along with my mood and my ability to make good choices or be nice to my traveling companion.

Most airports completely suck. Not to toot my own state's horn, but Portland's PDX is an exception — fresh scrambles, brown rice sushi, an assortment of salads, house-made soups, and made-to-order sandwiches on whole wheat bread. Way to go, Caper's Café. If you have a long flight ahead or a connecting flight and are forced to rely on airport food, opt for items that pack well, like turkey and avocado on a whole wheat bagel, raw nuts, and fruit. Avoid anything that won't stay fresh, like mayonnaise, so you don't end up lying on the teeny-tiny (and likely urinated on) floor of the plane's bathroom. Drink plenty of water always, but especially when you're traveling to keep you hydrated, maintain optimum metabolism, and prevent headaches.

It's almost not worth mentioning what tactic to take when you're on a plane these days, as hardly any airlines serve food in the coach cabin. The complimentary snacks like smoked almonds, peanuts, pretzels, and chips are all fatmakers and won't do much to satiate you. Do your best to avoid eating airline food in coach, even the meals you have to pay for. In first class, they tend to serve food that is a tad more palatable, but I've yet to see an airline serve sandwiches on whole wheat bread, and the egg and meat dishes are beyond scary.

CAMPING, BUSINESS TRIPS, VACATIONS, AND ROAD TRIPS

I hate camping. My parents completely ruined it for me during their hippie days when they quit their jobs, sold our house and all our belongings, bought a really crappy Volkswagen bus (which later caught on fire), and took four kids, ages two to seven, to Europe and Morocco for a year. Even though I was only five, I remember it vividly because it completely sucked and scared the H-E-Double-Hockey-Sticks out of me — which my parents found enormously amusing. We camped throughout Europe for months until we finally settled in a rental house in Fez, Morocco, that had lots of rugs but no furniture, which to me also felt like camping. (As a side note, if you like figs, go to Morocco, but don't put them in your pocket like my little brother did. It makes a huge mess and may really piss off your mom.) These days, you are not likely to find me on a camping trip.

Every few years, though, Cousin Helen from Canada decides we should have the family reunion at some hellish campground in Oregon. To me, this type of family gathering is a thinly veiled excuse to eat Doritos, s'mores, and hot dogs and drink cheap beer. As appetizing as this menu is to some of my relatives, I bring my own food. Oatmeal requires only boiling water. I also bring whole wheat rolls, canned tuna, raw almonds, raisins, fruit, veggies, homemade banana bread, and lots of wine. I have not trusted the wine to my Canadian family members since one torture-laden family reunion when Cousin Helen brought out huge jugs of cider wine. Not only does cider wine look less than appealing due to the weird things floating in the bottom of the jug; it also smells gross and tastes disgusting. As a bonus, it will leave you with a massive headache — so massive you would start writing your will if you could only hold a pen steady enough. Cousin Helen said I should have tried the peach "varietal" because she drank it and felt great! If you're coerced into camping, bring your own provisions, and put a snack in your pocket so you're armed with real fuel before they start passing around the Doritos at the family campfire.

I have to travel some for business, sometimes to real cities with real grocery stores and real restaurants, but sometimes I end up in particularly freakish places, like Gatlinburg, Tennessee. I've been there twice. It's a fake town set up to attract tourists and bears. As far as I could tell, Gatlinburg doesn't have any grocery stores. It does have all the caramel corn and cotton candy your heart desires, only it's bigger down there. If you're interested in salt and pepper shakers, you'll be delighted to know that Gatlinburg is the home of the world's only Museum of Salt & Pepper Shakers. Curiosity got the best of me, and I can proudly claim to have seen over twenty thousand different salt and pepper shaker sets. My favorites were the vegetable-shaped ones. Hard to make a leek very attractive, but you'd be surprised at how adorable the corn-on-the-cob shakers were. Gatlinburg does have a liquor store — which is cleverly disguised as a postal convenience store — so I wasn't totally screwed. I bought some wine and a set of postage stamps with cute little bears on them and drove around in search of a decent restaurant.

The restaurant choices weren't a total disaster. Mostly pancakes, waffles, and fried chicken, but they also had a Planet Hollywood. Under normal circumstances, you'd have to drag me in there kicking and shouting obscenities, but in this case, I was stuck making it my cafeteria for the week. At Planet Hollywood, even salads (unmodified) are full of fat, and the loud music — Abercrombie & Fitch loud — will make you want to scream. One day the soup was tomato, but usually they were serving something vile like cream of beer and mystery cheese. The other thing to avoid in the South is sweet tea. Holy Batcave, Robin! This tea is sweet, all right! When you're traveling for work, try your best to find a decent grocery store and a restaurant or two that serves food on the List.

When I'm on an actual vacation and not just a business trip, I want to immerse myself in another place, or perhaps even another culture. Totally doable. Eat Mexican food in Mexico, eat tapas in Spain, and eat weird foods with even weirder names in England. When I traveled to Italy, I broke a few of my own rules. You have to in Italy! You can't go all the way to Italy and not eat fresh bread and pasta (of the white variety... shhhh, don't tell anyone!) and not drink red wine with lunch *and* dinner. I did skip the gelato, ate very small portions, and ate fish and meat when I had the opportunity. But the most important thing I did — which I believe made all the difference — was that I walked everywhere. I was in Italy for a week and did not gain an ounce. Once you lose the fat, walking will become a true joy. I walked, ate, and drank my way through Italy, and I'd happily do it again!

On road trips, bring snacks for two reasons: you may not find anything for hours and hours, and if you do find something, it will probably be gross and not on the List. You also don't want to stumble on a restaurant when you are famished. Even if the place has a few decent options, someone you're traveling with may order a bacon double cheeseburger with large fries and a chocolate shake. And maybe that person will be your nine-year-old son and he won't be able to finish his entire meal because he's a child and kids tend to stop eating when they become full. So you'll have a bite of his leftover burger and then another, and pretty soon you will have polished it off, along with the rest of his fries and chocolate shake — and then you'll get to eat carrot sticks for dinner.

PLACES OF WORSHIP

I don't have a lot of religion. The Gray kids went to the highly unorthodox church of Steve and Kathryn. Our parents raised us with a wee bit of spirituality and an enormous amount of love, praise, affection, and chores. Sunday mornings consisted of

Dad making a giant egg scramble filled with leftovers from the fridge, followed by His Highness supervising his four obedient but completely annoyed children while we cleaned out the garage, pulled weeds, or washed the family cars. I'm not actually sure where Mom was. Every so often, my siblings and I would get curious about organized religion and want to attend church with one of our friends. This concerned our parents because they were sure we'd get sucked in and brainwashed, but they usually consented after we did a fair amount of begging and promising that we would only pretend we were listening. I tried many different denominations and discovered one common element: doughnuts.

I know many of you enjoy your weekly outing to be at one with your beliefs, but do doughnuts and sugar cookies really help to hit the message home? I'm all for congregating and sharing and becoming more enlightened people, but do your best to embrace the experience without fried, fattening, fake food. Join the refreshment committee and shake things up a bit by suggesting mini-bran muffins, oatmeal raisin cookies, and whole wheat blueberry scones instead.

Without a doubt, there are countless other places you may find yourself needing to eat; do your best to predict what your food options will be, and plan accordingly. The following are types of restaurants you may encounter or choose to patronize. I'm sure I've missed a few, but I'm confident that after reading the List, you'll know what to do.

SUSHI

Very few sushi restaurants offer brown rice rolls, and you don't eat white rice anymore, so now what? Sashimi! You think raw fish is gross? You're already eating it in your sushi rolls, unless you're ordering California rolls with "krab" meat, in which case, I'm begging you, please stop saying how much you just *loooove* sushi. What you love is fake crabmeat and white rice. You may as well be eating saltwater taffy. Sashimi is pure, buttery, lean fish that, when dipped in soy or ponzu sauce, melts in your mouth. I eat as much sashimi as I can afford. Your *fab*ulous friends will order Toro (fatty bluefin tuna belly) because they are so fabulous and they can, but I'm completely happy with Maguro (another type of tuna) or Hamachi (yellowtail) because these don't say "Market Price" (code for "Twice as Much as Everything Else") next to them. One way to ease into eating sashimi instead of rolled sushi is to ask your sushi chef to lightly sear the fish. He will undoubtedly be put out by this request, but it makes seafood taste slightly less fishy and allows you the chance to get used to eating raw fish without the buffer that white rice provides.

Make sure your favorite sushi restaurant uses the highest-quality fish possible, and don't be afraid to ask where your fish came from. "From our fish guy" is not an acceptable answer. I also eat miso soup, edamame (boiled and salted green soybeans), and a large salad. Edamame is an incredibly healthy snack — high in protein, high in fiber, low in fat, low on the glycemic index, full of vitamins, and rich in omega-3 fatty acids. They are easy to make at home too. The only caveat is soybeans are often genetically modified. Be bold and ask if your favorite Japanese restaurant is committed to providing their customers with non-GMO food.

Avoid anything that's been fried, like tempura (even the vegetable kind), and look out for things like fried shallots on salads and soups. Noodle dishes will likely contain soba noodles, which I mentioned earlier. They are made from buckwheat and wheat flour and are not a bad choice because of their high protein and low GI score, but I like to get some necessary fiber when I'm carb-loading, so at Japanese restaurants I skip the noodle dishes. You may also find an assortment of salads, like seaweed, cucumber, or oshitashi (spinach). Those are all good choices, provided the restaurant uses high-quality ingredients. Sake is rice wine and is fairly low in calories so is deserving of a spot on the List. I like mine cold and unfiltered.

MEXICAN

Ditch the white flour tortillas, the taco salad shells, the tortilla chips, and the gobs of cheese, and you can eat Mexican food; the more authentic, the tastier and better for you. Americans are to blame for Mexican food getting a bad rap. We added the cheese to tacos and the giant tortilla shell to taco salads. Flour tortillas are made with white flour and typically contain lard (animal fat). Sprouted, whole-kernel corn tortillas are your best option but are hard to find. Some grocery stores sell them, and authentic, non-American-style cantinas often make their own. They are whole grain and have very little fat and calories. Some restaurants also carry whole wheat tortillas, but these contain some form of oil to hold them together. Between white flour tortillas and whole wheat flour tortillas, I'll opt for whole wheat, but I'll choose whole-kernel corn above them both — steamed, not fried. An even better idea is to forego the giant calorie-laden flour tortillas and the corn tortillas altogether and order your burrito in a bowl. Fill your bowl with chicken, brown rice (a rare but lucky find), pinto or black beans, chunks of avocado, pico de gallo or salsa, and cilantro, and you've got a healthy Mexican meal that will fill you up, keep you going, and not compromise your fat-reducing efforts.

If your taco comes in a crispy shell, it has been fried. Skip anything crispy. That includes downing a bowl of chips and salsa before to your meal arrives. Crispy means more fat and calories. Meats marinated in sauces such as mole or salsa roja or verde are excellent choices. With Mexican food, the red or white sauce idea gets thrown out the *ventana*. You'll find plenty of red, but mole sauce is decidedly brown and is made with chilies, almonds, bitter chocolate, cinnamon, sesame seeds, raisins, cloves, onions, tomatoes, and chicken broth. It's pureed until smooth and is outstanding with chicken. Although there's nothing inherently unhealthy in it, it is fairly high in calories, which means just go easy or order your sauce on the side. Salsa roja (red) and verde (green) are blends of tomatoes, cilantro, chilies, onions, and other tasty and spicy additions. They are typically lowfat, low-calorie, and *muy delicioso*! Order some black or pinto — not refried — beans on the side. Refried beans are mashed with lard or oil so are much higher in fat and calories. Black or pinto beans cooked in broth are high in fiber and protein, low on the glycemic index, low in fat, and definitely on the List. Tortilla soup is also on the List, but hold the tortilla strips; it's so zesty and flavorful, you won't even miss them. So you can eat Mexican food, but you have to train yourself to see foods that are crispy, have gobs of cheese or sour cream, or are served with flour tortillas as foods that you don't eat.

And just a reminder: margaritas are not on the List. A Modelo Light or Corona Light is the perfect complement to Mexican food. So is a delicious glass of ice cold water. Stay away from aguas frescas. They are Mexican Kool-Aid, albeit with fresh fruit, but the high sugar content far outweighs the fresh fruit benefits.

And now for the million-dollar question. (Or *la pregunta del millón de dólares*. I took three years of high school Spanish for the sole reason that older students said we'd go on a bunch of field trips to Mexican restaurants. We did, but I'm not sure Portland, Oregon, was exactly the epicenter of authentic Mexican food in 1980. Most kids just ate hamburgers, but we had to order them in Spanish, which completely confused our servers. I digress again.) What about the guacamole?!? For me, the entire reason to eat Mexican food is for the guacamole or slices of avocado. It is not your enemy, but too much avocado can throw your efforts to reduce body fat off track. Eat it sparingly: no more than the equivalent of half a small avocado. Eat black olives sparingly as well. Remember, olives and avocados contain good fat, the kind your body needs in small doses. I love sour cream, but only the organic, lower-fat version is on the List, which means I eat it at home and not at Mexican restaurants. And I don't eat much, a tablespoon at best.

PIZZA

If pizza made with white crust is your only available option, hit the salad bar. Don't forget to pass on the croutons and go easy on the dressing and cheese. Some places offer whole wheat pizza crust. At those places, I pile mine with veggies and request a light amount of cheese. I may also add a lean meat like barbecued chicken if it's available. Gourmet pizzerias may have prosciutto, which is intensely flavorful, so a small amount does the trick. Prosciutto, caramelized onions, and goat cheese pizza with an olive oil–based sauce is a magical slice of paradise. Pepperoni and ground beef are high in fat and salt, so I avoid them completely. One nice big slice of whole wheat–crust pizza and a dinner salad with all the extras, and I am good to go. Flying Pie Pizzeria near my home in Portland has extra thin whole wheat pizza crust topped with organic ingredients, a decent wine selection, an arcade for the kiddies, and dozens of board games that you can play as long as you wish. Pizza perfection.

ITALIAN

Very few Italian ristorantes offer whole wheat pasta. This is disappointing because I truly love Italian food, especially the pasta dishes. If you get lucky and whole wheat pasta is available, don't forget to choose red over white when it comes to pasta sauce. Remember why? Of course you do: red sauces are tomato-based, while white sauces are cream-based and are consequently much higher in calories and fat. Pesto sauces and olive oil–based sauces are safe choices too, but they're typically higher in fat and calories than tomato-based sauces, so I ask for a light amount of sauce if I'm lucky enough to find whole wheat pasta dishes that include them. You are also likely to encounter meat-centered dishes, like chicken marsala or entrées with fish or steak. Veal, chicken, or eggplant Parmesan is heavily breaded (with white bread crumbs) so is best to avoid. Meat dishes are often accompanied with a starchy side, like pasta or maybe polenta. Have a salad instead, or ask for an extra helping of vegetables.

At a recent outing for Italian food, the menu was extensive and I settled on pork medallions in a tomato sauce with shitake mushrooms and broccoli rabe on the side. Not a bad choice — meat and vegetables in a tomato-based sauce. Totally on the List. The menu failed to mention that the broccoli was fried in tempura batter. Battered and fried food is most certainly not on the List. Minestrone soup would be an ideal selection for a side if it weren't loaded with white pasta.

Pass on the spumoni, gelato, and tiramisu too — all fat-makers. Savor a cup of lowfat or nonfat cappuccino or herb tea instead.

ITEM #16: EATING AWAY FROM HOME

STEAKHOUSES

Have a steak. Just skip the ribs, the bread, and the baked potato. Filet mignon, flank, circle, sirloin, and flatiron are the leanest options. Other cuts, like porterhouse or prime rib, are on the List, but eat them sparingly because their fat content can be up to four times as high as that of the leaner options. So eat a much smaller portion and be careful to cut off the fat. Try your best to frequent places that carry high-quality beef that is grass fed and free of hormones and antibiotics. Eat veggies or a salad on the side. Corn on the cob is fine too, but go easy on the butter.

THAI

Other than the white, starchy noodles and white rice, Thai food is relatively healthy. Go easy on coconut milk–based curry sauces and anything with cashews. When cooking Thai at home, I use light coconut milk. As I mentioned earlier, although coconut contains some saturated fat, it has healthy properties too. Some Thai restaurants offer brown rice even though you may not see it on the menu, so be sure to ask for it. Tom Ka Gai, or chicken coconut soup, or Tom Kha Kung, which has shrimp instead of chicken, is an excellent choice, and a shredded green papaya salad makes the ideal complement. I often start with an order of chicken satay with peanut sauce, which satiates me until my soup and salad arrive. Avoid anything fried, like spring rolls, wontons, or coconut shrimp. Salad rolls and summer rolls are not typically fried, but they're wrapped in white rice paper, so I either pass on them or consume only the healthy and delicious stuff inside.

CHINESE

Just say no to monosodium glutamate (MSG), white rice, and fried food. Your best bet is a chicken, shrimp, or tofu stir-fry, Szechuan chicken, or anything else that basically consists of meat and veggies. Sweet-and-sour dishes are loaded with sugar and usually come with breaded, fried meat. Barbecue pork is lean and makes an ideal choice. Egg drop soup is great, but ask for yours sans wontons. Egg rolls, spring rolls, and most Chinese appetizers are fried and not on the List. Of course, Americans are to blame for bastardizing Chinese food — on a recent trip to Hong Kong (although that's not exactly like visiting mainland China), I didn't encounter a single fried food.

FRENCH

A good French restaurant or bistro serves savory meats and seafood in fairly small portions. Rabbit, venison, and quail will likely be on the menu. If they aren't too gamey for you, go for it. Unlike your average chicken, game meats are naturally free-range, and venison contains essential omega-3 fatty acids. French restaurants have a bad rap because of all the butter they use in their sauces. Not much you can do once your savory meat entrée arrives at the table, so I focus on portion control, meaning, as much as I'd like to, I don't eat everything on my plate. Even though the portions are already petite and crazy expensive, eating a stick of butter is never a good idea. Be sure to skip the bread and order a salad right off the bat so you won't eat more of your entrée than you should. Ask for your salad to be tossed with a light amount of dressing. If your request is met with any attitude, just get the dressing on the side and try to toss it yourself. Broth-based soups like bouillabaisse (fish stew) or more elaborate seafood stews with clams, mussels, and assorted fish are a French-restaurant staple and a superb choice. If you like raw oysters, have at it. I think they're disgusting, but they certainly won't make you fat, unlike oysters that have been breaded and fried.

INDIAN

Indian food has so many good flavors and spices. Good Indian restaurants will offer long-grain basmati rice. You may also encounter barley or other whole grains. Watch out for fried or doughy foods. Go for meats and veggie dishes, and read through all the ingredients listed. Tandoori anything will typically be cooked over charcoal or a hot wooden fire. What results is smoky and flavorful and definitely on the List. It will probably be chicken, but I've seen shrimp and scallops served tandoori style as well. Don't be afraid to be a pain in the ass and ask questions about where the seafood comes from. If you're lucky enough to find red lentil–based dahl on the menu, go for it. It's got a bit of butter in it but also has coconut milk and lots of spinach. At least share some with your dining companion(s) and have a few bites. Yogurt-based sauces are pure perfection, but go easy on the creamy and oily ones. If you encounter whole grain naan (Indian flatbread), definitely try a piece, but stay away from the far more common white versions. It's easy to overeat at Indian restaurants, so watch your portions and the amount of sauces or condiments you add to your meat and side dishes.

GREEK

Some excellent options. I love Greek sauces and dips, like tzatziki (yogurt-based), hummus (garbanzo bean–based), and melitzano (eggplant-based). What I'm usually lacking at a Greek restaurant is an acceptable dip-delivery vehicle. You're unlikely to find whole grain bread or pita. An alternative is to order some meat, seafood, or sliced cucumbers to mop up your dip with. Eat feta cheese and kalamata olives in small doses. Avoid casseroles, things made with phyllo dough, items wrapped in grape leaves, and layered appetizers and entrées. Gag me with a spoon, but if you're feeling adventurous, try some octopus marinated in olive oil, vinegar, and garlic. I prefer fasolia giahni (aka gigantes), which are beans baked in tomato sauce. Gyros are basically Greek fast food. I like the contents of gyros, which is typically rotisserie meat, tomatoes, onions, and tzatziki sauce; I just don't eat the white pita shell they come with. I'm pretty confident the meat is not up to my standards, so I limit gyros to no more than once a year. Broth-based and lentil-based soups are a terrific choice. Traditional Greek salads usually include feta cheese, kalamata olives, tomato, cucumber, and raw onions tossed in olive oil — an ideal choice, but go easy if you're also ordering a lamb, pork, or chicken entrée. You'll have plenty of meat choices, like souvlaki (meat kababs); just skip the potatoes and rice that typically accompany them. You may be tempted to try a glass or shot of ouzo, an anise-flavored liqueur. Ouzo is basically sugar and alcohol and is not on the List. If you're actually on a Greek island, have a celebratory sip, but at your average Greek restaurant, stick with wine or water.

MIDDLE EASTERN

I only learned of Middle Eastern food a few years ago, and I'm a huge fan. My favorite dish is vegetarian kibbe, which resembles a pâté and is made from bulgur (cracked wheat) mixed with fresh tomatoes, basil, mint, and onions. You're likely to find falafel (vegetable patties or balls made from garbanzo beans, parsley, onions, cilantro, and spices), which are often served with pita bread, tahini (sesame seed based) sauce, and tomatoes. If by some stroke of luck you encounter whole wheat pita bread, make yourself a small but tasty falafel sandwich. Baba ghanoush is another savory dish, consisting of roasted eggplant mixed with tahini sauce, lemon juice, and garlic and typically served with olive oil and pita bread. Tabbouleh (finely chopped parsley, bulgur, tomatoes, mint, and green onions, mixed with olive oil and lemon juice), lentil soups, and meat kababs are other good choices. Middle Eastern food is pretty healthy fare, but it's also a bit high in calories. Watch your portions, go easy on sauces, feta cheese, and olives, and pass on white pita bread and refined rice.

MEDITERRANEAN

Hard to go wrong. You'll find plenty of meats and vegetables, soups, salads, and starters that are on the List, like lamb kababs, roasted beet salad, grilled shrimp or scallops, braised beef, and seafood stew. Avoid refined versions of rice, polenta, and pasta. Skip the bread. You'll encounter plenty of cheeses, olives, and fried dishes like calamari. I would pass on the cheese, enjoy a few olives, and (for all eternity) avoid fried dishes of any kind. Mediterranean appetizers can be wonderful — roasted beets and arugula with small pieces of blue cheese, and ahi tuna with avocado are two of my favorites. Sorry, those little crostinis (tiny cheese toasts) that come with many starters are not on the List.

SPANISH AND TAPAS

Be on the lookout for breaded items, white rice dishes, and egg dishes with pastry shells. Tapas can very quickly add up the calories. It's best to find one vegetable-based dish, like green beans or a salad, and one protein-based dish, like fava beans, meatballs, or seared scallops, and call it good. Sangria is made with wine, but it also has fruit juice in it. Find a Spanish red or white wine to complement your meal instead.

BURGER JOINTS

Slim pickins here. The culprit is the white bun. The French fries and milkshakes are also a problem. I keep saying I'm going to smuggle in my own whole wheat bun and switch it with the white one. I've yet to do this, but someday I'll get bold enough if the burger is really worth it. Otherwise, sorry, you need to train yourself to go bunless, but you'll have "less bun" as a result! (Bet you're wishing I'd have "less pun.") Beef burgers are okay once in a while, but choose buffalo, turkey, grilled chicken, or meatless burgers if they are available. I'm a big fan of buffalo burgers. Buffalo meat contains omega-3s, is lower in fat and higher in protein than beef, and tastes amazing. Whatever you decide, it's best to load your burger up with all the extras: Dijon mustard, ketchup, dill pickles, lettuce, tomatoes, red onions, and a couple slices of avocado. Steer clear of the mayo and cheese, and make sure all your condiments, like ketchup and mustard, are certified organic so you're not loading up on HFCS. Every so often, I'll throw in a slice or two of nitrate-free bacon, but only when I can "afford" it — not the monetary cost, but the cost to my waistline. Maybe you're the adventurous type and would enjoy grilled pineapple, sprouts, sautéed mushrooms and onions, or poblano peppers on your burger. All those items are a-okay.

When a real beef burger craving strikes you, do your best to find a hamburger joint that serves high-quality grass-fed beef that was raised without hormones or antibiotics. And train yourself to steadfastly believe that you do not eat French fries under any circumstances. Or potato chips — no one can eat just one, so don't try the one-bite method here. I've been using the List as my food guide for an awfully long time and I really trust myself, but not with French fries or potato chips. Broken record here: fill up on salad or a cup of soup instead.

DELIS AND CAFÉS

Though they're hard to come by, I thoroughly enjoy a good deli. I include cafés with delis because minus the deli case of cheese and meat and jars of gross things that resemble floating eyeballs, they have very similar offerings. Turkey on whole wheat with all the fixins and a cup of split pea soup is lunch perfection in my mind. Train yourself to make it a habit to order your sandwich without mayo and cheese. If you add mayo and cheese, the Denim Diet says you only get half a sandwich. I personally would rather eat the whole darn thing, but your choice. No negotiating on potato or macaroni salad. School cafeterias have disgusting coleslaw; good delis have delicious coleslaw — the chunkier, the better, and the sauce should be a bit runny and not just resemble mayonnaise. Fortunately, this type of gourmet coleslaw is on the List.

HAPPY HOUR

Typical bar and happy-hour food can make you fat. It is rare for me to find more than one or two items on the menu that I will eat. Sometimes I get lucky, and grilled scallops, tuna tartare, Caesar salad, or roasted beets will be on the menu. I'm not trying to be a total smartass here, but the nicer the restaurant, the better your options are going to be. There are a few restaurants in Portland that I can patronize only at happy hour because it's the only time I can afford them. The Heathman Hotel is one example. Their chef, Philippe Boulot, is a James Beard Award winner, which to me means I can't afford eating at his restaurant. The bar menu, however, is awesome and super-reasonable, offering Caesar salad, crab cakes, and deviled eggs. I happen to think the bar is considerably more charming than the hotel restaurant, which is stuffy and, well, hotel-like.

And don't forget what's on the List when it comes to alcohol. Cocktails and mixed drinks will sabotage your progress and can make you fat. Take it easy on alcohol, and drink water to slow you down, keep you hydrated, and ensure your ability to exercise sound judgment. Almost any time is a good time for a glass of water.

BUFFETS

Call me a snob if you want. I use the term *barf-fets* because I can't tell you how many times I've been to a buffet when someone in my party threw up afterward — starting with my sister in 1976, in the Kmart parking lot after eating at North's Chuck Wagon. Aside from losing your brunch, the big problem with buffets is eating more than one plateful or piling too much on your plate. If you must eat at a barf-fet, survey your choices and figure out what you are going to eat before you start piling anything on your plate, and limit your meal to a few items that are on the List. Maybe an omelet with fruit, carved turkey with green beans and salad, or smoked salmon with scrambled eggs and whole wheat toast — one of those platefuls, not all three.

COSTCO, TARGET, AND IKEA

Huge shocker here, but Costco dogs are not on the List. Neither are 90 percent of all the little samples that are scattered throughout the store. I never go to Costco on an empty stomach, and neither should you — or your children if you're forced to tote them along. I can't stand shopping at Costco, but I know many people are addicted to it, and the store does carry an array of items that are on the List — nuts, fruit, vegetables, meats, wine, spaghetti sauce, coffee beans, whole wheat bread, and a surprisingly extensive (and growing!) list of organic choices.

In general, eateries in big-box stores like Costco, Target, and Ikea offer food that is low in quality, high in fat, high in sodium, and best to stay away from. Sweden-based Ikea has some bizarre menu items, but there are a couple of decent choices, like the green herbed salmon (without the dill sauce) and the vegetarian sandwich on whole wheat bread. The twenty-meatball plate with gravy and boiled potatoes, however, is not on the List. Did you know that one Ikea meatball has thirty-five calories and over two grams of fat? Eating the twenty-meatball plate? You do the math! Feel like a little snack while shopping at Target? Brace yourself. The nachos at Target contain 1,101 calories, fifty-six grams of fat, and 66 percent of the recommended daily allowance for sodium.

7-ELEVEN

Convenience stores are good for gossip mags, toilet paper, lottery tickets, wine (in a pinch), and protein bars, in that order. Okay, you can include feminine hygiene products in that list, but for real food, find a decent grocery store or a farmers' market.

VENDING MACHINES

You can't read the labels through the Plexiglas, so even protein bars aren't a good option. Candy bars are not on the List. Neither are pretzels, potato or corn chips, sweetened trail mixes, granola bars (most contain HFCS), chewing gum (neither sugary nor artificially sweetened), or peanut butter cracker sandwiches. Save your quarters for laundry or poker night.

When choosing a restaurant or any establishment that serves food, look for a place that serves organic, local, and seasonal ingredients that are raised or grown using sustainable methods. It won't be too difficult to determine — restaurants tend to brag about such things, and rightly so. When possible, avoid chain restaurants. These typically have low-quality choices that are high in fat, calories, and, sodium and offer little in the way of real nutrition. I realize that in some parts of the country, dining out healthfully is easier said than done, and I've been spoiled rotten by the outstanding chefs and restaurant choices in Portland. I don't expect that many of you are sushi chefs or care to make your own whole-kernel corn tortillas, but plenty of the suggestions that I've provided in this section can also be applied to cooking meals at home. The recipes in the back of the book can help get you started.

ITEM #16: EATING AWAY FROM HOME

1. Try using FPV (Food Planning and Visualization) before you eat out. Reading restaurant menus online helps a lot!
2. Eat a healthy snack before going to dinner parties, office parties, birthday parties, and baby or bridal showers.
3. Avoid specialty cocktails with sugary mixers.
4. Load up on salad and veggies at dinner parties.
5. Use the "two-thirds veggies, one-third protein" rule for your dinner plate.
6. Skip dessert, cake, and punch at all parties unless, of course, you are the guest of honor.
7. If you're going to a potluck, bring a dish that's on the List.
8. Bring your own snacks to entertainment venues.
9. When possible, avoid airport and airplane food.
10. Bring your own food when you go camping.
11. Find a decent grocery store or restaurant when you're on a business trip.
12. Relax a bit on vacations, but walk more to balance out your indulgences.
13. Keep some healthy snacks on hand for road trips.
14. Weekly worship needn't include doughnuts or cookies.
15. Before you head out to eat, consult the restaurant sections in this chapter so you're armed with a few ideas of what to look for on the menu.
16. Save your quarters for poker or laundry night and never use them for vending machines.

FOOD BLISS

THERE IS A RESTAURANT BY MY HOUSE called Laughing Planet. They have an item on their menu called Soylent Green. It is served hot in a bowl and contains chunks of chicken breast (or tempeh for vegetarians), shitake mushrooms, barley, quinoa, Swiss chard, and broccoli with a shitake mushroom sauce. It's a large bowl of pure goodness. I feel good when I eat it. I eat every last bite and feel energized and satisfied. I feel like I did something good for my body, and it makes me happy.

That may sound strange, and maybe you can't imagine in your wildest dreams that you could be overjoyed about a dish called Soylent Green, but I love it. I hope you learn to experience this kind of food bliss. Your food bliss will likely be derived from a different dish altogether, maybe even one that you've concocted yourself. I hope someday you will see wholesome, nourishing food like this as a beautiful thing and a privilege to eat.

Once you learn to place your emphasis on purposeful eating and your goal in eating becomes maximum health and reaching and maintaining your ideal, healthy body weight, dishes like Soylent Green taste amazing. There are times when I order something that sounds like it has Food Bliss potential but when it arrives I see that I couldn't have been more mistaken. Not long ago, I ordered the kaiso salad at a local sushi restaurant. It had five kinds of seaweed, fresh crab, and cucumber slices in lemon juice and sweet vinegar. How unpleasant could it be? Very. It was slimy and gross, and I could tell my dining companion felt sorry for me as he demolished a dozen giant sauce-laden white-rice sushi rolls one after the other. I just smiled and happily chomped away at my kaiso salad, knowing that while it wasn't exactly a taste sensation, it met my criteria for healthful eating. When I woke up the next morning, I reflected on how good I felt. I was full of energy, I had slept well, my skin was clear, I hadn't compromised my health by eating foods that don't meet my standards, and I could still get into my favorite pair of jeans. I won't order that salad again, but no regrets here. That particular restaurant has a bunch of great menu items, like sashimi, and next time I'll be less adventurous.

Even when you're at home, sit down to eat. Take your time. Savor each bite and visualize all the good things your food is doing for your body. See every bite of your meal being used to your benefit. Realize how awesome it is that you get to enjoy plentiful, delicious food and that it's not making you fat. It may taste a little different from what you're used to, but you'll easily develop a taste for it.

Most important, be kind to yourself. Learn to love your

body. Loving your body will help you make good decisions. The List is not a hard-core philosophy for having a fit, healthy body or for being a better steward of our amazing planet. It's a balanced approach, and I believe in it. Moreover, I don't believe in overly strict diets and doing without. I want my cup of coffee in the morning. It smells good, tastes good, and goes superbly with the daily crossword puzzle. I also don't value being super-skinny. I'm cranky and look like death when I don't weigh enough. Eat, but eat well. I have complete faith in you and believe in the strength and power of your mind, and I wish you well on your journey.

THE DENIM DIET SUMMARY

THE LIST	HABITS TO MAKE	HABITS TO BREAK
1. Sweeteners	• Purified water • Coffee or tea • Raw brown sugar, honey, agave nectar • Syrups: barley malt, brown rice, maple • Stevia • Not adding sweetener (best) • Trusting your instincts (your gut)	• Diet or regular soda pop • Sports drinks or energy drinks • High fructose corn syrup (HFCS) • White pure cane sugar • Splenda, Sweet'N Low, NutraSweet, Equal • Overdoing it on any sweetener • Trusting the corn refiners and beverage companies
2. Carbohydrates	• Whole grains: wheat, kamut, spelt, oat, barley, rye • Brown rice, whole wheat couscous, chia, quinoa • Whole grain pasta • Whole-kernel corn or whole wheat tortillas • Sweet potatoes • Fruit, veggies, beans, lentils, seeds • Low-glycemic, high-fiber carbs	• White, processed, refined grains • White rice, white couscous • White (semolina) pasta • White flour tortillas • White potatoes • Brownies, cake, pie, gummy bears, etc. • High-glycemic, low-fiber carbs; high-protein diets
3. Eating Organic	• Certified organic; fair trade if possible • Buying in bulk • Buying local at farmers' markets and co-ops; checking labels at grocery store • Cast-iron, stainless steel, or baked-enamel pans	• Foods made using conventional methods; GMOs • Buying packaged, processed foods • Regularly buying from giant agribusiness manufacturers • Teflon/nonstick pans

4. Fast Food	• Drastically limiting consumption of fast food • Grilled chicken, whole wheat buns, organic beef • Keeping healthy snacks in your car on road trips • Soup and salad; easy on the dressing, no croutons	• Consuming fast food on a regular basis • HFCS, trans fat, saturated fat • Being overly hungry when dependent on fast food • Taco salad shells, white buns, fried food, milkshakes
5. Alcohol	• 1 or 2 drinks a day, a few days per week • Red or white wine, light beer • Hard alcohol straight or with water or club soda • Eating before and/or while you drink — olives, nuts, whole wheat crackers, etc.	• Daily consumption of alcohol • Microbrews • Cocktails, blended or mixed drinks • Skipping snacks to avoid calories when drinking alcohol
6. Caffeinated Drinks	• Regular coffee (2–5 cups maximum/day), decaf, or tea • Half-and-half, lowfat milk, or skim milk • Unsweetened or with sweeteners from Item #1	• Foo-foo coffee milkshakes — mochas, flavored lattes, Frappuccinos, etc. • Presweetened liquid or powder creamers • White sugar or artificial sweeteners
7. Breakfast	• Eating breakfast every morning • Eating breakfast at home; ditching the café pastries, muffins, and bagels • Whole wheat pancakes, French toast, and waffles; easy on the maple syrup and butter • Skim or lowfat plain organic yogurt • Whole grain cereals with few ingredients, unsweetened or with sweeteners from Item #1 • Scrambled, poached, or hard-cooked eggs • Low-saturated fat, vitamin D–fortified dairy; small doses of butter and cream	• Skipping breakfast • Pastries and other breakfast foods at cafés like Starbucks • White-flour pancakes, French toast, and waffles; fake maple syrup • Presweetened yogurt • Cereals with HFCS, trans fat, or white sugar • Eggs Benedict, quiche, cheesy omelets • Regular/extensive use of butter and cream

THE DENIM DIET SUMMARY (CONTINUED)

THE LIST	HABITS TO MAKE	HABITS TO BREAK
7. Breakfast (continued)	• Fruit- or veggie-only smoothies; limiting juice • Eating fruit as your breakfast side dish	• Large, sugar-filled smoothies; excessive juice • Eating hash browns or cottage fries as your breakfast side
8. Protein	• Eating red meat once a week or less • Grass-fed, antibiotic- and hormone-free beef • Lean meats: chicken, fish, buffalo, bison • Vegetarian protein sources such as legumes, seeds, and nuts • Eating only Eco-Best seafood	• Excessive amounts of red meat • Grain-fed, antibiotic- and hormone-filled beef • Excessive amounts of pork and lamb • Contributing to world hunger and starvation by consuming excessive beef • Eating seafood that's high in mercury and toxins or that destroys habitats
9. Fruits and Veggies	• 5–9 servings of colorful fruits and vegetables daily • Roasting vegetables in heart-healthy oils, such as olive, canola, or walnut	• Drowning vegetables in sauces, creams, butter, or dressing • Fried (tempura) vegetables
10. Good Fats	• Checking cholesterol levels — LDL, HDL, and triglycerides • Unsaturated fats: canola, peanut, and olive oil; omega-3s: flax, salmon, and tuna	• Thinking you're too young to worry about cholesterol • Excessive saturated fats; trans fats; believing that eating fat makes you fat

11. Going Green	• Reusable grocery bags • Real, raw, whole foods • Finding ways to reduce your carbon footprint • Buying "new-to-you" stuff	• Plastic or new paper bags • Packaged, prepared foods • Complacency, helplessness, inaction • Buying new stuff
12. Snacking	• Eating when you're hungry • Small, high-protein, low-glycemic snacks • Snacking at midmorning or midafternoon • Watching sodium intake; using sea salt	• Waiting it out until the next meal • Snacking on sweets, cookies, or processed foods • Snacking at midnight • High-sodium, processed, prepared food
13. Exercising	• Minimum of 30 minutes of daily walking or other exercise • Taking stairs; walking to errands; stretching daily; weightbearing exercise 3 times weekly	• Maintaining weight without heart-healthy movement • Getting stuck in routine/not mixing it up to maintain interest and decrease boredom
14. Food Enablers	• Sticking to your plan with friends and family • Modifying your meals from what others are eating, if necessary	• Caving in to "well-meaning" food enablers • Taking care of your family's health but not yours
15. Portions and Calories	• Setting limits on calories; deck of cards–size portions • Keeping a health journal — calories, diet, exercise	• Large portions and mindless snacking • Obsessing over daily weigh-ins
16. Eating Out	• Finding restaurants that serve local, sustainable, organic food • Meal planning using online menus; snacking before dinner parties	• Eating at chain restaurants • Showing up at restaurants or dinner parties overly hungry/unprepared

STOCKING THE PANTRY

NOW THAT YOU'RE ALL READY TO PUT THE LIST IN ACTION and practice new habits to get your energy up and your waistline down, how about a little headstart on what to stock the refrigerator and pantry with? First, you might want to do a little housekeeping. Put your reading glasses on because you'll need to check out those labels and be on the lookout for ingredients like high fructose corn syrup and trans fats! Credit for the following grocery store list goes to WholeFoods.com, but I made a few modifications so it's 100 percent List-approved. Happy shopping!

FRUITS AND VEGGIES BY COLOR

- Red: Strawberries, cherries, raspberries, apples, tomatoes, watermelon, radishes
- Orange: Sweet potatoes, pumpkin, cantaloupe, oranges, grapefruit, peaches, carrots
- Yellow: Pineapple, bananas, yellow squash, mangoes, bell peppers

- Green: Spinach, kale, chard, green beans, green peas, zucchini, snow peas, bell peppers, kiwis
- Purple/blue: Grapes, eggplant, plums, blackberries, blueberries, açaí berries

WHOLE GRAINS

- Whole grain and sprouted grain bread, rolls, English muffins, pita pockets, and so on
- Whole wheat and whole-kernel corn tortillas
- Whole wheat pasta
- Brown rice, bulgur, quinoa, chia, wheat berries, brown basmati rice, wild rice, whole wheat couscous
- Whole wheat crackers
- Whole grain cereals and oats

PROTEIN: MEAT AND SEAFOOD

- Nitrate-free deli meats
- Chicken, pork, turkey, buffalo, lamb, or beef
- Chicken, turkey, and pork sausage
- Canned tuna (dolphin safe)
- Assorted fresh fish and seafood

PROTEIN: DAIRY

- Milk or unsweetened soy or rice milk
- Soy cheese, cottage cheese, lowfat sour cream

- Light string cheese, Parmesan cheese, mozzarella cheese
- Plain yogurt (nonfat or lowfat)

PROTEIN: BEANS, EGGS, NUTS, SEEDS

- Beans: dry and canned, including black, pinto, navy, garbanzo (chickpeas), lima, fava, white
- Soy-based tofu and tempeh
- Eggs
- Natural nut butters (peanut and almond)
- Raw almonds, peanuts, pecans, pistachios, walnuts, Brazil nuts, hazelnuts
- Seeds: flax (ground), pumpkin, sunflower, sesame

A LITTLE SOMETHING SWEET

- Applesauce (no added sugar)
- All-fruit jams and jellies
- Dark chocolate — with 70 percent or higher cocoa content

BASIC STAPLES

- Oils: olive, canola, flaxseed, walnut, peanut, sunflower, soybean, hempseed, corn (check labels, as some oils require refrigeration)
- Seasonings: sea salt, black and cayenne pepper, fresh and dried herbs and spices
- Condiments: ketchup (HFCS-free), mustard, hummus, hot sauce, balsamic vinegar, apple cider vinegar, salsa

- Sweeteners: agave nectar; raw honey; raw cane sugar; barley, rice, and maple syrups; stevia
- Baking ingredients: flaxseed meal, wheat germ, whole wheat flour, molasses, vanilla extract, almond extract

BEVERAGES

- Coffee: regular or decaf
- Tea: black, green, oolong, and herb
- Red or white wine
- Light beer
- Club soda or sparkling water as mixer for hard alcohol drinks

KAMI'S TOP TEN TRIMMING TIPS

S INCE I DRESS PEOPLE FOR A LIVING, it would seem a shame
not to pass along some surefire ways for instantly looking
five pounds thinner. (These are mostly for women, but men can
benefit from many of them as well.)

1. WEAR CLOTHES THAT FIT YOU. Your tops, bottoms, and
   undergarments should not be too small or too large. Over-
   sized clothing adds weight and makes you look like you're
   trying to hide in your clothes. Undersized clothing squeezes
   the top layer of subcutaneous fat (which we all have to some
   extent) and creates a muffin top, fatback, and peek-a-boo
   breasts. A good bra that provides proper coverage is essential to tops and blouses fitting correctly.

2. WEAR DARK COLORS ON BOTTOM, LIGHT COLORS ON TOP.
   White and light colors add weight, and dark colors subtract
   weight. For most people, the bottom half is larger, so to create the illusion of it being less pronounced, wear dark jeans,
   pants, skirts, and shorts and pair them with lighter tops.

3. **LAYER ON TOP.** It's hard to get away with much when wearing a single layer on top — every little bump shows. Pair lightweight tops, blouses, polos, tanks, and tees with cardigans, blazers, hoodies, or a second T-shirt. Make sure that whatever top(s) you wear covers the midriff when you reach for something or blow-dry your hair. A long, completely opaque camisole or tank top worn tucked or untucked can be layered under almost everything.

4. **ADD SOME HEIGHT.** Routinely wearing high heels can wreak havoc on your back and posture, but occasionally a little boost to your height can create a dramatic difference. Someone 5'6" and 145 pounds looks 5'10" and the same exact weight when wearing a pair of four-inch boots or heels. Make sure your pant hem almost reaches the floor to create the longest-looking legs possible.

5. **FORGO EMBELLISHMENTS.** Ribbons, bows, jewels, and other adornments dangling from your clothes add bulk and make people around you dizzy. Simple, classic, solid fabrics create the most slimming look.

6. **DO DENIM RIGHT.** Jeans should not be too short — they should almost reach the floor. Make sure your jeans have back pockets; pocket-free jeans don't look good on any body type. If you have a muffin top (that is, more fat around your midriff), get a larger size or choose a different brand or style. Jeans that come up too high on the waist create the appearance of a long behind. Bootcut jeans have by far the most flattering hem type; narrow hems are for skinny,

trendy, young people. Also, the darker the denim, the more flattering, and no pleats in front!

7. **USE SELF-TANNER OR BRONZER FOR PALE LEGS.** If you weren't blessed with naturally tan or dark skin, adding a bit of color to your legs when wearing shorts, skirts, or dresses works like magic to slim and even tone your legs. Bronzer also hides spider veins and other unsightly blemishes. However, it smells horrible, so apply it at night and rinse it off in the morning. Try Physicians Formula Organic Wear 100% Natural Origin Liquid Bronzer.

8. **MAKE SURE YOUR SLEEVES AND STRAPS FIT.** The sleeve opening should fit around the circumference of your arm and not be too tight. For tank tops, make sure the straps are loose enough that extra skin is not oozing on either side of them. Sleeve lengths that cover down to the elbow look the most flattering.

9. **CHOOSE THE RIGHT SHOES.** Wear shoes that create a low contrast with what you're wearing on the bottom. For example, pairing black shoes with black pants, tan shoes with bare legs, or brown or rust shoes or boots with denim will create a more flattering, lengthy, cohesive appearance than wearing a pair of bright red pumps with your jeans.

10. **WEAR BLACK.** Nothing does the trick better than black. So you don't look funeral bound, wear a colorful scarf around your neck or some fun but tasteful jewelry.

DENIM DIET RECIPES

by Kelly Ballew

NOW THAT YOU'VE ADOPTED Kami's approach to healthy eating, here are some recipes for you to try. In the ingredient lists, although I recommend that all ingredients be certified organic, I add the word *organic* only for certain items, like soy flour and cornstarch, that would likely otherwise be made from GMOs.

In the breakfast section, we've got your bases covered whether you're in the mood for savory or sweet. The egg dishes can be cooked as scrambles or frittatas, and you can cut cholesterol, fat, and calories without sacrificing much flavor by reducing the number of egg yolks. We've included recipes for List-approved brunch cocktails along with two of the scrambles. Check out the Baked Goods section for List-approved breakfast pastries as well as healthy dessert options for special occasions.

The sandwiches, wraps, soups, and salads are so filling, flavorful, and beautiful, you'll want to serve them not just for lunch but for dinner and Sunday brunch too. You can add meat or seafood to many of the recipes to make the dishes even more substantial. If you do, be sure to select certified-organic meats and Eco-Best seafood.

BREAKFAST DISHES

Hearty Hotcakes

The first time I made these for my kids, they either didn't notice they were eating whole grain pancakes or they were so happy to have a hot breakfast that they didn't complain. Either way, they gobbled them up, and so did I.

Makes about twelve 5-inch pancakes

1 cup whole wheat flour
¼ cup organic soy flour
¼ cup flaxseed meal
¼ cup buttermilk powder
1 teaspoon baking soda
1 teaspoon baking powder
½ teaspoon ground cinnamon
¼ teaspoon sea salt
3 large egg whites, beaten
1 tablespoon expeller-pressed organic canola oil, plus more for brushing
1½ cups nonfat or lowfat milk (more or less depending on desired thickness)
2 teaspoons amber agave nectar
½ teaspoon vanilla extract
1 cup fresh or thawed frozen blueberries (optional)
Warmed maple syrup for serving

In a large bowl, combine the flours, flaxseed meal, buttermilk powder, baking soda, baking powder, cinnamon, and salt. Whisk to blend. In a medium bowl, combine the egg whites, the 1 tablespoon oil, the milk, agave nectar, and vanilla extract. Whisk to blend. Add to the dry ingredients and stir until just blended; do not overmix.

Heat a griddle or a large skillet over medium-low heat and brush with canola oil. Pour the batter into a pitcher, then pour a 5-inch-diameter circle of batter for each pancake. If using blueberries, sprinkle a few on top of each circle of batter after you pour it. Cook until bubbles appear in each pancake and the bottom is golden brown, 3 to 5 minutes. Flip over with a spatula and cook on the other side for 1 to 3 minutes. Keep pancakes warm in an oven on low heat while cooking the remaining batter. Serve with maple syrup.

VARIATIONS: Substitute banana slices for the blueberries. Or top finished pancakes with nut butter and warmed raw honey or agave nectar.

Quinoa Porridge

Have you noticed how often there is a bowl of porridge in fairy tales? It's warm, tasty, and — dare I say? — magical. Double or triple the recipe on Sunday morning, and you'll be eating like a queen or king all week. You can reheat the leftover porridge in a small saucepan on the stovetop, or in the microwave.

Makes 4 servings

½ cup quinoa
1 cup water
1¾ cups nonfat milk
1 cup old-fashioned rolled oats
⅓ cup chopped dried apples
⅓ cup raisins
½ teaspoon sea salt
½ cup plain nonfat yogurt
2 tablespoons amber agave nectar
1 tablespoon flaxseed meal
1 tablespoon toasted wheat germ
1 teaspoon ground cinnamon
¼ cup chopped raw almonds or hazelnuts

Place quinoa in a fine-mesh strainer, rinse thoroughly with cool water, and drain. In a small saucepan, combine the quinoa and water and bring to a boil. Reduce the heat to a simmer, cover, and cook until all water is absorbed, 10 to 15 minutes.

In a medium saucepan, bring the milk to a simmer over medium heat. Stir in the oats, apples, raisins, and salt. Reduce the heat to low, cover, and cook for 3 minutes. Stir in the cooked quinoa and cook until heated through, 1 to 2 minutes. Remove from the heat and stir in the yogurt, agave nectar, flaxseed meal, wheat germ, and cinnamon. Serve divided among 4 cereal bowls, sprinkled with the nuts.

Yumi Yogurt

As opposed to Yami? Get it? Kami's love of play-on-words has officially rubbed off on me. Forget those presweetened yogurts. Serve this version for breakfast, a midmorning snack, lunch, or dessert. It's quick and especially good with fresh, seasonal berries in the summer. In case you don't like cinnamon, I list it as optional, but keep in mind that it's a superfood that lowers blood sugar, triglycerides, LDL (or bad) cholesterol, and total cholesterol.

Makes 4 servings

2 cups plain nonfat yogurt
2 teaspoons amber agave nectar
¼ teaspoon vanilla extract
¼ teaspoon ground cinnamon (optional)
½ cup mixed fresh berries
2 tablespoons chopped raw almonds or walnuts, or a mixture of
   the two
2 teaspoons flaxseed meal (optional)
2 teaspoons toasted wheat germ (optional)

In a medium bowl, combine the yogurt, agave nectar, vanilla extract, and optional cinnamon. Stir gently to blend. Divide among 4 bowls and top with the berries and nuts. For extra fiber, omega-3s, and crunch, sprinkle with flaxseed meal and wheat germ, if you like.

Mediterranean Scramble

It's tough to go wrong with a scramble. Almost anything savory can be paired with eggs. Kami and I grew up with our dad's Sunday-morning scrambles made from refrigerator leftovers. This one is colorful and appetizing, and the combination of feta cheese, olives, and spinach is delicious and ridiculously good for you.

Makes 4 servings

8 large eggs, or 6 large eggs and 4 large egg whites
2 tablespoons half-and-half
2 tablespoons nonfat milk
¼ cup crumbled feta cheese
¼ cup finely chopped black or Greek olives
½ cup chopped plum tomatoes
1 cup chopped spinach
½ cup finely chopped red onion
2 to 3 tablespoons minced fresh basil
1 clove garlic, minced
½ teaspoon freshly ground black pepper
½ teaspoon sea salt
1 tablespoon olive oil

In a large bowl, combine the eggs, half-and-half, and milk. Whisk to blend. Add all the remaining ingredients except the oil and stir to blend. In a large skillet, heat the olive oil over low heat and pour in the egg mixture. Let set for a minute before gently stirring until the eggs are cooked. Divide among serving plates and serve at once.

MEDITERRANEAN FRITTATA: In a large skillet, heat the oil over medium-high heat. Reduce the heat to medium, pour in the scramble mixture, and cover. Cook for 10 to 15 minutes, or until nearly set. Finish the frittata by putting a plate over the pan, inverting the frittata onto the plate, and then sliding it back into the pan to cook the other side. Or place the pan (which should be ovenproof) under a broiler for 1 to 2 minutes. Serve now, or let cool completely. Cut into wedges to serve, or use as a sandwich filling. Makes 4 servings.

South-of-the-Border Scramble

Serve as a summer supper with baked whole grain corn tortilla "chips" and salsa. A mojito (recipe follows) is *muy fantastico* with this spicy egg dish.

Makes 4 servings

8 large eggs, or 6 large eggs and 4 large egg whites
2 tablespoons half-and-half
2 tablespoons nonfat milk
¼ cup shredded extra-sharp Cheddar cheese
1 small avocado, peeled, pitted, and diced

½ cup cherry tomatoes, halved
¼ cup chopped green onions, including green parts
1 red bell pepper, seeded, deveined, and diced
2 tablespoons minced fresh cilantro
1 (4-ounce) can peeled green chilies, drained and chopped
¼ cup organic salsa
½ teaspoon sea salt
½ teaspoon freshly ground black pepper
1 tablespoon Cilantro-Lime Dressing (page 266; optional)
1 tablespoon olive oil

In a large bowl, combine the eggs, half-and-half, and milk. Whisk to blend. Add all the remaining ingredients except the oil and stir to blend. In a large skillet, heat the olive oil over low heat and add the egg mixture. Let set for a few seconds, then gently stir until the eggs are cooked. Divide among serving plates and serve at once.

SOUTH-OF-THE-BORDER FRITTATA: In a large skillet, heat the oil over medium-high heat. Reduce the heat to medium, pour in the scramble mixture, and cover. Cook for 10 to 15 minutes, or until nearly set. Finish the frittata by putting a plate over the pan, inverting the frittata onto the plate, and then sliding it back into the pan to cook the other side. Or place the pan (which should be ovenproof) under a broiler for 1 to 2 minutes. Serve now, or let cool completely. Cut into wedges to serve, or use as a sandwich filling. Makes 4 servings.

Mojito

Makes 2 drinks

2 ounces fresh spearmint leaves
2 teaspoons amber agave nectar
2 ounces white rum
10 ounces club soda
Juice of 1 fresh lime, plus 2 lime wedges for garnish
Crushed ice

In a pitcher, combine all the ingredients except the lime wedges, and stir with a spoon to crush the mint leaves. Pour into 2 tall glasses. Serve at once with a lime wedge on the rim of each glass.

Garden Walnut Scramble

If you've never given succulent green beans and eggs a try, you're in for a treat. Serve for your next Sunday brunch and be prepared for rave reviews. For celebratory occasions, serve with a simplified Bellini (recipe follows).

Makes 4 servings

3 tablespoons olive oil
1 pound green beans, trimmed and cut into bite-size pieces
½ cup finely chopped yellow onion
2 cloves garlic, minced

5 ounces cremini mushrooms, chopped
¼ cup chopped walnuts or whole pine nuts
8 large eggs, or 6 large eggs and 4 large egg whites
2 tablespoons half-and-half
2 tablespoons nonfat milk .
¼ cup grated Parmesan cheese, plus more for serving
1 tablespoon minced fresh flat-leaf parsley
1 tablespoon minced fresh basil
½ teaspoon sea salt
½ teaspoon freshly ground black pepper, plus more for garnish
Sautéed chicken-apple sausage slices, cut into bite-size pieces
    (optional)

In a large sauté pan, heat 1 tablespoon of the olive oil over medium heat. Add the green beans and sauté until tender, approximately 6 to 8 minutes. Reduce the heat slightly and add 1 tablespoon olive oil. Add the onion, garlic, mushrooms, and nuts and sauté until the onion is translucent, about 3 minutes. Remove from the heat and set aside.

In a large bowl, combine the eggs, half-and-half, and milk. Whisk to blend. Add the green bean mixture, the ¼ cup cheese, the parsley, basil, salt, pepper, and sausage, if using. Stir to blend. In a large skillet, heat the remaining 1 tablespoon olive oil over low heat and add the egg mixture. Let set for a few seconds, then stir until the eggs are cooked. Divide among serving plates and serve at once, sprinkled with more Parmesan and ground pepper.

GARDEN WALNUT FRITTATA: In a large skillet, heat the 1 table-spoon oil over medium-high heat. Reduce the heat to medium, pour in the scramble mixture, and cover. Cook for 10 to 15 minutes, or until nearly set. Finish the frittata by putting a plate over the pan, inverting the frittata onto the plate, and then sliding it back into the pan to cook the other side. Or place the pan (which should be ovenproof) under a broiler for 1 to 2 minutes. Serve now, or let cool completely. Cut into wedges to serve, or use as a sandwich filling. Makes 4 servings.

Bellini

Makes 1 drink

4 ounces sparkling wine or champagne
1 slice fresh nectarine or apricot
1 or 2 fresh raspberries

Pour the wine into a champagne flute. Add the fruit and serve.

BAKED GOODS

Coffee Spice Cake

A delicious complement to your morning cup of coffee or tea. Spread the goodness — coffee cake is easy to share. Bring a batch to work, your book club, your next family brunch, or a church social. Throw some shaved dark chocolate on top and serve with Sweet Yogurt Cheese Spread (recipe follows), and you've got the perfect special-occasion dessert.

Makes one 9-inch square cake; serves 9

2½ cups whole wheat flour
¼ cup organic soy flour
¼ cup flaxseed meal
¼ cup toasted wheat germ
¼ cup whey protein powder
1 teaspoon baking soda
1 teaspoon baking powder
½ teaspoon sea salt
3 teaspoons ground cinnamon
½ teaspoon ground ginger
¼ teaspoon ground cloves
¼ teaspoon ground nutmeg
1 cup buttermilk, or 1 cup milk with 1 tablespoon fresh lemon
    juice
½ cup amber agave nectar or raw honey

1 large egg, or 2 large egg whites
¾ cup plain nonfat yogurt
2 tablespoons unsalted butter, melted, or ¼ cup unsweetened
    smooth applesauce
1 teaspoon vanilla extract
2 tablespoons organic brown sugar

Preheat the oven to 350°F. Brush a 9-inch square baking pan
with canola oil.

In a medium bowl, combine the whole wheat flour, soy flour,
flaxseed meal, wheat germ, protein powder, baking soda, baking powder, salt, 2 teaspoons of the cinnamon, the ginger,
cloves, and nutmeg. Whisk to blend. In a large bowl, combine
the buttermilk, agave nectar, eggs, yogurt, butter, and vanilla
extract. Whisk until smooth. Add the dry ingredients to the wet
ingredients and stir until just blended; do not overmix. Pour the
batter into the prepared pan and smooth the top.

Stir the remaining 1 teaspoon cinnamon and the sugar together
in a small bowl. Sprinkle evenly over the top of the batter.

Bake in the center of the oven for 30 to 35 minutes, or until a
toothpick inserted in the center of the cake comes out clean.
Remove from the oven and let cool completely in the pan. Cut
into squares.

Sweet Yogurt Cheese Spread

Makes ¾ cup

1 cup plain nonfat yogurt
2 rounded teaspoons agave nectar
1 teaspoon ground cinnamon
½ teaspoon vanilla extract
¼ teaspoon almond extract

Line a colander with 2 layers of dampened cheesecloth. Place the colander over a bowl and empty the yogurt into the colander. Cover and refrigerate for at least 6 hours. (The longer the yogurt drains, the thicker it will become.) Stir in the agave nectar, cinnamon, vanilla extract, and almond extract. Cover and refrigerate for at least 1 hour and up to 3 days.

Energy Bars

Okay, soccer moms — this one's for you! Forget the packaged, processed granola bars doled out at the end of the game. Show the team how much you love them by fueling them up with some real, wholesome food made with raisins, dried fruit, oats, and whole wheat flour. This recipe is sweetened with agave nectar, which means your darling kids won't get a spike in their blood sugar level and drive you nuts on the way home from the game. When enjoying these bars for breakfast or snacking at home, serve with Sweet Yogurt Cheese Spread (above).

Makes 8 bars

1 teaspoon expeller-pressed organic canola oil
1¼ cups old-fashioned rolled oats
¼ cup toasted wheat germ
¼ cup whole wheat flour
¼ cup flaxseed meal
¼ cup amber agave nectar
1 large egg white
2 tablespoons plain nonfat yogurt
2 teaspoons unsulphured dark molasses
1 teaspoon vanilla extract
⅓ cup raisins or chopped dried apples or apricots, or a
   combination
1 teaspoon ground cinnamon
½ teaspoon sea salt
⅓ cup dark chocolate chips (optional)

Preheat the oven to 300°F. Brush an 8- or 9-inch square baking pan with canola oil.

In a large sauté pan, heat the oil over low heat, add the oats, and toast, stirring frequently, for 10 minutes. Pour the oats into a large bowl.

Add to the oats all the remaining ingredients and stir until mixed. Spread the mixture in the prepared pan and press down firmly and evenly using an oiled rubber spatula. Bake in the center of the oven for 18 to 20 minutes, or until lightly browned. Remove from the oven, let cool completely, and cut into bars to serve.

Power Pumpkin Bread

This is not your average pumpkin bread. Packed with protein and fiber, it's dense, filling, and especially good toasted and thinly spread with almond butter or hazelnut butter, or served as a dessert, with Sweet Yogurt Cheese Spread (page 236).

Makes two 8-by-4-inch loaves (sixteen 1-inch slices)

½ cup raisins (optional)
2 cups whole wheat pastry flour
½ cup organic soy flour
½ cup whey protein powder or nonfat milk powder
¼ cup oat bran or wheat bran
½ cup toasted wheat germ
½ cup flaxseed meal
1 ½ tablespoons baking powder
1 teaspoon ground cinnamon
½ teaspoon ground nutmeg
½ teaspoon ground cloves
½ teaspoon ground ginger
½ teaspoon salt
3 large eggs, or 2 large eggs plus 2 large egg whites
1 (15-ounce) can pumpkin puree
¾ cup plain nonfat yogurt

½ cup unsweetened smooth or chunky applesauce
1 tablespoon unsulphured dark molasses
1 cup shredded zucchini
1 cup shredded carrots
½ cup raw almonds, chopped

Preheat the oven to 350°F. Brush two 8-by-4-inch loaf pans with canola oil and dust with flour; knock out the excess flour. Soak the raisins (if using) in boiling water to cover for 15 minutes, then drain.

In a large bowl, combine the flours, protein powder, oat bran, wheat germ, flaxseed meal, baking powder, cinnamon, nutmeg, cloves, ginger, and salt. Whisk to blend. In a large bowl, beat the eggs until frothy. Add the pumpkin, yogurt, applesauce, and molasses. Stir until blended, then stir in the zucchini and carrots. Gradually stir in the dry ingredients until just blended. Fold in the nuts and raisins.

Pour into the prepared pans, smooth the tops, and bake in the center of the oven for 1 hour, or until a toothpick inserted in the center of the bread comes out clean. Remove from the oven and let cool on wire racks for 10 minutes. Unmold onto the racks and let cool completely. Cut into slices to serve.

VARIATIONS: This bread can be made without the zucchini and carrots. Buttermilk powder can be used in place of the protein powder or dry milk powder; add 1 teaspoon baking soda to the dry ingredients. Other chopped nuts or ground seeds can replace the almonds, and chopped dried fruits, such as apricots, pears, cherries, or cranberries, can be used in place of the raisins.

Apple Banana Bread

Banana bread is almost foolproof and lends itself well to a whole grain version with a rich, nutty goodness. Toast or microwave a slice, spread it thinly with hazelnut or peanut butter, and enjoy it with your coffee or tea for breakfast. Banana bread is also good with Sweet Yogurt Cheese Spread (page 236).

Makes one 9-by-5-inch loaf; serves 10 to 12

1 cup whole wheat flour
¼ cup organic soy flour
¼ cup flaxseed meal
2 teaspoons baking powder
½ teaspoon sea salt
¼ cup expeller-pressed organic canola oil
¼ cup unsweetened chunky applesauce
½ cup amber agave nectar
2 tablespoons unsulphured dark molasses
1 large egg plus 2 large egg whites, beaten
3 very ripe bananas, mashed (2 cups)
1 teaspoon vanilla extract
⅓ cup chopped walnuts or raw almonds
1 cup raisins

Preheat the oven to 325°F. Grease a 9-by-5-inch loaf pan with canola oil and dust with flour; knock out the excess flour. Soak the raisins in boiling water to cover for 15 minutes; drain.

In a medium bowl, combine the flours, flaxseed meal, baking powder, and salt and whisk to blend. In a large bowl, combine the oil, applesauce, agave nectar, and molasses and stir until blended. Stir in the eggs, bananas, and vanilla extract. Gradually stir in the dry ingredients until blended. Fold in the nuts and raisins. Scrape into the prepared pan and smooth the top.

Bake in the center of the oven for 1 hour to 1 hour and 15 minutes, or until a toothpick inserted in the center of the bread comes out clean. Remove from the oven and let cool completely in the pan. Cut into slices to serve.

VARIATION: Add ½ cup mini–dark chocolate chips. Spread with Sweet Yogurt Cheese Spread (page 236).

ABC Crisp

This apple-blackberry-cranberry crisp is as easy as its name indicates. It sounds like a dessert and would make an excellent candidate, but it's so chock-full of good things that it's an ideal breakfast choice as well. Leave the peels on the apples, as most of the vitamins and much of the fiber is in the peels. The almond extract in the yogurt topping gives this recipe a surprising flavor twist.

The DENIM DIET

Makes one 9-by-13-inch crisp; serves 12

FILLING

6 unpeeled tart apples, such as Braeburn, Pink Lady, or Fuji,
  cored and thinly sliced
2 cups fresh or frozen blackberries
½ cup dried cranberries
2 tablespoons whole wheat flour
1 teaspoon ground cinnamon
¼ cup amber agave nectar

CRUMBLE

½ cup old-fashioned rolled oats
½ cup whole wheat flour
1 tablespoon flaxseed meal
1 tablespoon toasted wheat germ
1 teaspoon ground cinnamon
2 tablespoons organic brown sugar
4 tablespoons cold unsalted butter
¼ cup finely chopped nuts

TOPPING

1 cup plain nonfat yogurt
½ teaspoon vanilla extract
¼ teaspoon almond extract
1 tablespoon raw honey

Preheat the oven to 350°F. Lightly butter a 9-by-13-inch baking dish.

FOR THE FILLING: Spread the apples evenly in the prepared dish. Layer with the blackberries and cranberries. In a medium bowl, combine the flour and cinnamon and stir to blend. Sprinkle over the fruit. Drizzle evenly with the agave nectar.

FOR THE CRUMBLE: In a medium bowl, combine the oats, flour, flaxseed meal, wheat germ, cinnamon, and brown sugar and stir. Cut the butter into the dry mixture with a pastry cutter until coarse crumbs form. Stir in the nuts.

Sprinkle the crumble evenly over the filling. Bake in the center of the oven for 30 to 40 minutes, or until the apples are tender and the crumble is golden brown. Remove from the oven and let cool slightly.

FOR THE TOPPING: In a small bowl, combine all the ingredients and stir until blended.

Serve in shallow bowls with a spoonful of topping.

VARIATION: Substitute fresh raspberries or fresh or frozen blueberries for the blackberries, or use a combination of the three kinds of berries.

Berry Turnovers

These can be served for either breakfast or dessert. They're wholesome and filling to start the day, but they're also perfect drizzled with melted dark chocolate as a snack. Hint: Tell your kids they're homemade Pop Tarts.

Makes 6 turnovers

1 cup whole wheat pastry flour
¼ teaspoon sea salt
3 tablespoons expeller-pressed organic canola oil
¼ teaspoon vanilla extract
¼ teaspoon almond extract
3 tablespoons water
2 teaspoons amber agave nectar
Milk for brushing
½ cup 100 percent fruit spread or crushed fresh berries

In a medium bowl, combine the flour and salt. Whisk to blend. In a small bowl, combine the oil, vanilla extract, almond extract, water, and agave nectar. Stir the wet ingredients into the dry ingredients until evenly moistened. On a floured board, form the dough into a ball. Cover in plastic wrap and refrigerate for 1 hour.

Preheat the oven to 350°F. Brush a baking sheet with canola oil and dust with flour; knock out the excess flour.

On a floured board, use a rolling pin to roll the dough into an 8-by-12-inch rectangle and cut into six 4-inch squares. Roll each square into a 5-inch square. Brush the edges of each square liberally with milk (to seal). Place 1 rounded tablespoon of fruit spread on one side of each square and spread, leaving a ½-inch rim on all sides. Fold the pastry over the fruit spread. Press the edges together with a fork.

Place the turnovers on the prepared pan and bake in the center of the oven for 15 minutes, or until golden brown. Remove from the oven and let turnovers cool slightly on a wire rack. Serve warm or at room temperature.

SANDWICHES AND WRAPS

Fiesta Salsa Wraps

Anything with avocado gets my full attention. These wraps shine in spring and summer, when fresh vegetables abound. The combination of avocado with corn and sweet peppers is a delicious way to pack antioxidants, fiber, vitamins, minerals, and much more into a single dish.

Makes 6 wraps

FIESTA SALSA
Makes approximately 4 cups (leftover salsa can be stored in an airtight container in the refrigerator for up to three days)

¾ cup canned pinto or black beans, drained and rinsed
1 small yellow onion, finely diced
1 small red bell pepper, seeded, deveined, and finely diced
1 medium avocado, peeled, pitted, and diced
½ teaspoon grated lime zest
Juice of 2 limes
½ cup fresh, canned, or frozen corn kernels
2 Roma tomatoes, finely diced
3 cloves garlic, minced
2 green onions, chopped, including green parts
½ teaspoon freshly ground black pepper
¾ teaspoon sea salt

1 tablespoon minced fresh cilantro

¼ teaspoon ground ginger

½ teaspoon ground cumin

¼ teaspoon chili powder or more to taste

1 teaspoon minced fresh oregano

WRAPS

12 8-inch whole wheat or whole-kernel corn tortillas

½ cup lowfat sour cream

Juice of 1 lime

1 teaspoon minced fresh cilantro

Lightly seared ahi tuna chunks, thin strips of roasted chicken
    breast, or poached wild salmon in small chunks (optional)

Leaves from 1 head romaine lettuce, shredded

FOR THE SALSA: In a medium bowl, combine all the ingredients
and stir to blend. Cover and refrigerate for at least 2 hours or up
to 3 days.

FOR THE WRAPS: Preheat the oven to 300°F. Wrap the tortillas
in aluminum foil and heat in the oven for about 5 minutes.

In a small bowl, combine the sour cream, lime juice, and cilantro.
Stir to blend.

Spread approximately ½ cup salsa in a line across the bottom
third of a tortilla. Top with a little of the sour cream mixture and
the tuna, chicken, or salmon, if using, then with some shredded

lettuce. Fold over the filled part of the tortilla, then fold in the sides and proceed to fold the tortilla the rest of the way. Repeat to use the remaining tortillas and fillings. Serve at once.

FIESTA SALSA SALAD: Serve ½ cup salsa on a bed of the shredded lettuce and top with the sour cream mixture and optional meat.

Hummus Harvest Pitas

These beautiful dinner party appetizers have something for everyone. Guests love to stack assorted vegetables on top of the hummus and pita wedges to make mini-sandwiches.

Serves 6 to 8 as an appetizer

HUMMUS
¾ cup water
¾ cup tahini (sesame paste)
4 to 6 cloves garlic, minced
Juice of 3 lemons
1 tablespoon olive oil
¼ teaspoon freshly ground black pepper
¾ teaspoon ground cumin
½ teaspoon sea salt
2 (15-ounce) cans garbanzo beans, drained and rinsed

PITAS AND ACCOMPANIMENTS

4 whole wheat pita pockets, each cut into 6 wedges

Sliced unpeeled or partially peeled cucumbers

Grape, cherry, or sliced plum tomatoes

Finely chopped green onions, including green parts

Pitted kalamata olives

Crumbled feta or goat cheese

Red bell pepper strips

FOR THE HUMMUS: In a blender, combine all the ingredients and puree until smooth. Cover and refrigerate for at least 2 hours or up to 5 days.

TO SERVE: Place the hummus in a serving bowl in the center of a large platter. Arrange the pita wedges and accompaniments neatly on the platter and serve.

VARIATIONS: Cut each pita bread in half instead of into wedges, and tuck some hummus and accompaniments inside for a meal-size version. Or spread the hummus on large lettuce or spinach leaves, add some vegetables, and roll up for a wrap.

Cucumber Sandwiches

A healthier and more filling version of the little sandwiches traditionally served for high tea. For heartier appetites, roast turkey is an ideal complement to the cucumber and yogurt. The spicy yogurt cheese spread is also excellent on whole wheat crackers, slices of whole grain naan, or pita wedges, served as an appetizer.

Makes 6 sandwiches

6 whole wheat pita pockets, halved
Spicy Yogurt Cheese Spread (recipe follows)
1 English cucumber, thinly sliced (about 3 cups)
2 tablespoons finely chopped red onion (optional)
Sliced roast turkey breast (optional)

Spread some Spicy Yogurt Cheese Spread in each pita pocket half. Add about ¼ cup cucumber slices as well as optional ingredients, if you like.

Spicy Yogurt Cheese Spread

Makes approximately 1 cup

1⅓ cups plain nonfat yogurt
1 clove garlic, minced
1 tablespoon grated Parmesan cheese
⅛ teaspoon ground cumin

¼ teaspoon red pepper flakes
¼ teaspoon sea salt
¼ teaspoon freshly ground black pepper
1 tablespoon minced fresh basil
1 tablespoon minced dry-packed sun-dried tomatoes

Line a colander with 2 layers of dampened cheesecloth. Place the colander over a bowl and empty the yogurt into the colander. Cover and refrigerate for at least 6 hours to make yogurt cheese. (The longer the yogurt drains, the thicker the yogurt cheese will be.)

In a food processor or blender, combine the yogurt cheese, garlic, Parmesan cheese, cumin, red pepper flakes, salt, and pepper. Puree until smooth. Fold in the basil and sun-dried tomatoes. Cover and refrigerate for at least 1 hour and up to 3 days.

Spicy Bean Burgers

Since most soy burgers and "garden" burgers are over-processed and full of sodium, GMOs, and fake ingredients, it's well worth the time to make your own. These can be enjoyed alone or on top of Fiesta Salsa Salad (page 248), with Cilantro-Lime Dressing (page 266). To serve as sandwiches, use whole grain buns and top with your choice of avocado, Dijon mustard, organic ketchup, sliced tomato, and/or sliced red onion.

Makes 6 patties

½ cup quinoa

1 cup water

2 (15-ounce) cans pinto or black beans (or a combination), rinsed and drained

½ cup fresh or thawed frozen corn kernels

⅓ cup Fiesta Salsa (page 246) or store-bought organic salsa

⅓ cup finely chopped red onion

¼ cup finely chopped dry-packed sun-dried tomatoes

1 (4-ounce) can peeled green chilies, drained

2 cloves garlic, minced

1 large egg, beaten

1 large egg white

¼ teaspoon red pepper flakes

½ teaspoon ground cumin

½ teaspoon sea salt

¼ teaspoon freshly ground black pepper

1 tablespoon olive oil

Place quinoa in a fine-mesh strainer, rinse thoroughly with cool water, and drain. In a medium saucepan, combine the quinoa and water. Bring to a boil, reduce the heat to a simmer, cover, and cook until the water is absorbed, 10 to 15 minutes.

Puree the beans in a food processor or with a ricer until smooth, or put them in a bowl and mash them with a potato masher. Combine the pureed beans, quinoa, and all the remaining ingredients except the oil and stir well to blend. Shape into six 4-inch patties.

In a large skillet, heat the olive oil over medium-high heat. Add the patties and sauté until browned, about 4 minutes on each side.

Egg Salad on Flatbread

As an alternative to store-bought breads like whole grain sandwich bread, pita bread, whole wheat tortillas, or whole-kernel corn tortillas, try making your own flatbread. Things just taste better when you make them yourself. I've offered an easy egg salad topping suggestion, but any number of things can be eaten with these healthy crackerlike breads.

Makes 4 open-face sandwiches

FLATBREAD
¾ cup whole wheat flour
¼ cup organic soy flour
¼ cup flaxseed meal
½ teaspoon sea salt
¼ cup water, plus more as needed
1 tablespoon olive oil, plus oil for brushing

EGG SALAD
4 hard-cooked large eggs, chopped
4 hard-cooked large egg whites, chopped
2 to 3 tablespoons Mock Mayonnaise (page 255) or lowfat
    mayonnaise

1 tablespoon minced fresh chives or green onion
1 tablespoon finely chopped celery
1 tablespoon minced fresh parsley
1 tablespoon minced fresh oregano
1 tablespoon minced fresh thyme
1 teaspoon Dijon mustard
¼ teaspoon cayenne pepper
½ teaspoon sea salt
½ teaspoon freshly ground black pepper
Paprika for dusting (optional)

FOR THE FLATBREADS: In a large bowl, combine the flours, flaxseed meal, and salt. Whisk to blend. Stir in the ¼ cup water and the 1 tablespoon olive oil. Add 1 or 2 teaspoons water if needed to make a moist dough. On a floured board, knead the dough until smooth. Divide into 4 balls and use a rolling pin to roll each ball into a flat oval about 6 inches long.

Brush a large sauté pan with olive oil and heat over medium-high heat. Cook each flatbread until golden brown, 1 to 3 minutes per side. Keep warm in an oven on low heat while cooking the remaining flatbreads.

FOR THE EGG SALAD: In a medium-size bowl, combine all the ingredients.

Spread each flatbread with about ½ cup egg salad. Dust with paprika, if desired, and serve.

Mock Mayonnaise

Mayonnaise is obviously not a meal in itself (although Kami made up an extremely repetitive and annoying song when she was in fourth grade about wishing the world were made of mayonnaise), but we're including this recipe because store-bought mayo and even mayo alternatives are highly processed and high in calories and fat. This recipe provides a great alternative without the guilt.

Makes about 1 cup

1 cup water
1 tablespoon organic cornstarch
2 tablespoons olive oil
1 tablespoon apple cider vinegar
2 tablespoons plain nonfat yogurt
1 teaspoon Dijon mustard
¾ teaspoon sea salt

In a small saucepan, whisk the water and cornstarch together. Place over medium heat and whisk constantly until the mixture comes to a boil. Cook, whisking constantly, for 3 to 5 minutes, or until the mixture is almost clear.

Pour into a medium bowl and whisk in the remaining ingredients one at a time. Let cool completely. Refrigerate in a tightly sealed container for up to 1 week.

SOUPS AND SALADS

Cream of Pumpkin Soup

This healthier version of creamy pumpkin soup will help take the autumn chill off. Serve with a colorful Farmers' Market Salad (page 263) and a crusty whole wheat baguette, and you have the perfect fall dinner.

Makes 8 servings

1 tablespoon unsalted butter
1 large yellow onion, chopped
6 cups vegetable broth
2 (15-ounce) cans pumpkin puree
2 teaspoons amber agave nectar
¼ cup half-and-half
½ teaspoon ground cinnamon
¼ teaspoon ground cloves
¼ teaspoon paprika
½ teaspoon ground ginger
1 tablespoon minced fresh thyme
1 teaspoon sea salt
1 cup plain nonfat yogurt, plus 8 tablespoons
¼ cup minced fresh chives
Paprika and ground cinnamon for dusting

In a soup pot, melt the butter over medium heat and sauté the onion until translucent, about 3 minutes. Add 1 cup of the vegetable broth; bring to a boil, then cover, reduce the heat, and simmer for 15 minutes. Puree in a blender until smooth. Return to the pot and add the remaining 5 cups vegetable broth, the pumpkin, agave nectar, half-and-half, cinnamon, cloves, paprika, ginger, thyme, and salt. Bring to a boil, cover, reduce the heat to a simmer, and cook for 15 minutes, stirring occasionally. Add the 1 cup yogurt, whisk vigorously, and simmer for 5 minutes. Do not boil.

Ladle into individual bowls and top each serving with a tablespoon of yogurt. Sprinkle each serving with chives and dust with paprika and cinnamon.

Roasted Tomato Seafood Stew

You could use almost any combination of seafood in this zesty stew. A crusty whole wheat baguette is a must to have on hand for dipping and soaking up every last bite. For more festive occasions, finish off with a dollop of crabmeat, some lowfat sour cream, and a pinch of chopped chives placed in the center of each bowl before serving.

Makes 8 servings

2 tablespoons olive oil

1 large yellow onion, diced

8 cloves garlic, minced

1 tablespoon minced fresh thyme

1 tablespoon minced fresh basil

1 tablespoon minced fresh oregano

1 teaspoon sea salt

1 teaspoon freshly ground black pepper

1 (28-ounce) can fire-roasted tomatoes

¼ cup tomato paste

2 stalks celery, sliced

2 tablespoons ketchup

1 tablespoon Worcestershire sauce

2 teaspoons organic soy sauce

Dash of hot sauce

8 cups vegetable broth

1 pound salmon, skin and pin bones removed

1 pound steamer clams, scrubbed

1 pound jumbo shrimp, shelled and deveined (tails intact)

6 to 8 fresh basil leaves, coarsely chopped

¼ cup grated Parmesan cheese

In a large sauté pan, heat the oil over medium heat and add the onion, garlic, thyme, basil, oregano, salt, and pepper. Sauté until the onion is translucent, about 3 minutes.

In a blender, combine half of the tomatoes with the tomato paste, celery, ketchup, Worcestershire sauce, soy sauce, hot sauce, and onion mixture. Puree until almost smooth. Pour the mixture into a soup pot. Puree the remaining tomatoes in the blender and pour into the pot along with 1 cup of the vegetable broth. Bring to a boil, then add the remaining 7 cups vegetable broth. Reduce the heat to a simmer and cook for 1 hour. Add the salmon and clams and cook for about 5 minutes, or until the salmon is opaque and the clams have opened. Add the shrimp and basil. Simmer for 2 to 3 minutes, or until the shrimp are evenly pink. Ladle into stew bowls and sprinkle with Parmesan; serve.

Three-Bean and Ham Soup

As much as I loved Campbell's Bean with Bacon Soup as a kid, now that I realize what's in it, like sodium nitrate and monosodium glutamate (MSG), I like my version a lot better. Be sure to use certified-organic (nitrate-free) ham. Serve as a light supper with Crunchy Cobb Slaw (page 262), a good loaf of whole grain bread, and a glass of Oregon Pinot Noir.

Makes 8 servings

1 (15-ounce) can white beans
1 (15-ounce) can black beans
1 (15-ounce) can pinto beans
1 tablespoon olive oil
1 yellow onion, chopped
2 cups chopped 1-inch-thick ham steak (about 1 pound)

6 cups water

3 vegetable bouillon cubes

2 teaspoons whole wheat flour

½ cup wheat berries

1 cup brown rice

½ cup chopped celery

2 carrots, peeled and sliced

2 tablespoons minced fresh flat-leaf parsley

Drain the beans, reserving ¼ cup of the broth from one of the cans. Rinse the beans and set aside.

In a soup pot, heat the olive oil over medium heat and sauté the onion for 3 minutes, or until translucent. Add the ham and sauté another minute or two. Add the water and bouillon cubes. Bring to a boil, reduce the heat to a rapid simmer, and stir until the bouillon dissolves. Stir the flour into the reserved bean broth. Whisk the flour mixture into the soup and cook, whisking constantly, for 2 or 3 minutes. Add the rinsed beans, wheat berries, rice, celery, and carrots and cook for 15 minutes. Reduce the heat to a low simmer. Add the parsley and cook for about 45 minutes longer, or until the rice and wheat berries are cooked and the stew is flavorful.

VARIATION: If you prefer a thinner soup, omit the flour and discard the reserved bean broth.

Turkey and Spinach Soup

Spinach adds a wallop of healthy goodness to this hearty soup. Rosemary, the secret ingredient, contributes its own special fragrance. Serve with crusty whole wheat bread and a glass of Sauvignon Blanc.

Makes 8 servings

2 tablespoons olive oil
1 yellow onion, chopped
1 clove garlic, minced
2 cups chopped carrots
8 cups vegetable broth
1 tablespoon minced fresh thyme
1 tablespoon minced fresh oregano
1 tablespoon minced fresh rosemary
1 teaspoon sea salt
½ teaspoon freshly ground black pepper
2 (15-ounce) cans white beans, rinsed and drained
3 cups diced cooked turkey breast
1 bunch spinach, stemmed and rinsed, or 1 (10-ounce) package
    thawed frozen chopped spinach

In a large soup pot, heat the olive oil over medium heat and sauté the onion, garlic, and carrots until softened, about 5 minutes. Add the vegetable broth, thyme, oregano, rosemary, salt, pepper, beans, and turkey. Bring to a boil, cover, reduce the heat to a simmer, and cook for 20 minutes. Remove from the heat and stir in the spinach until wilted. Ladle into bowls and serve immediately.

Crunchy Cobb Slaw

I'm taking a few liberties with the name *Cobb*, but this crunchy slaw will get you right on track for your daily dose of fiber and antioxidants. It's so colorful and filling that it can be served on its own for lunch. A home-brewed iced green tea with lemon slices would make this a health-packed home run.

Makes 8 main-course servings

2 boneless, skinless chicken breast halves
1 unpeeled crisp apple, such as Braeburn, Pink Lady, or Fuji, cored and coarsely chopped
1 cup finely chopped red cabbage
3 carrots, peeled and shredded
1 cup finely chopped cucumber
¼ cup finely chopped red onion
¼ cup finely chopped green onion, including green parts
¼ cup raisins
2 tablespoons fresh lemon juice
¼ cup plain nonfat yogurt
½ teaspoon sea salt
½ teaspoon freshly ground black pepper
1 rounded teaspoon raw honey
3 fresh mint leaves, minced

⅓ cup Gorgonzola cheese
¼ cup slivered almonds

In a medium saucepan, bring about 3 inches of salted water to a boil. Add the chicken, reduce the heat to a simmer, and cook until the chicken is opaque throughout, approximately 6 to 8 minutes. Remove from the heat, drain (reserve the cooking liquid for soup), and let cool to room temperature. Cut the chicken into 1-inch cubes and set aside.

In a large bowl, combine the apple, cabbage, carrots, cucumber, red onion, green onion, raisins, and 1 tablespoon of the lemon juice. Toss to mix. In a small bowl, combine the yogurt, the remaining 1 tablespoon lemon juice, the salt, pepper, honey, and mint. Stir to blend. Add the yogurt mixture to the apple mixture and toss. Add the chicken and cheese and toss again. Cover and refrigerate for at least 1 hour or up to 2 hours. Fold in the almonds just before serving.

Farmers' Market Salad

Serve this celebration of vegetables as a first course or to accompany a sandwich or a bowl of soup. Feel free to make substitutions depending on what's fresh where you live. A simple balsamic vinaigrette can be substituted for the raspberry dressing.

Makes 6 first-course or side-dish servings

5 cups mixed baby greens
1 cup finely chopped red cabbage
2 chopped plum tomatoes
1 large red or orange bell pepper, seeded, deveined, and diced
½ cup thinly sliced carrot
1 cup sugar snap peas, trimmed and halved crosswise
1 unpeeled Granny Smith apple, cored and coarsely chopped
¼ cup raw almonds, chopped, or whole pine nuts
¼ cup shredded extra-sharp Cheddar cheese
Raspberry Vinaigrette (recipe follows)
½ cup fresh raspberries
3 hard-cooked large eggs, thinly sliced (optional)

In a large bowl, combine the greens, cabbage, tomatoes, bell peppers, carrots, snap peas, apple, nuts, and cheese. Toss with the raspberry vinaigrette. Divide among salad bowls or plates and top each serving with raspberries and optional egg slices.

Raspberry Vinaigrette

Makes approximately ⅔ cup

¼ cup olive oil
¼ cup raspberry vinegar
1 tablespoon plain nonfat yogurt
1 tablespoon lowfat sour cream
1 teaspoon agave nectar

1 teaspoon dry mustard
½ teaspoon sea salt
¼ teaspoon freshly ground black pepper

In a blender or a jar with a tight-fitting lid, combine all the ingredients and blend or shake until combined.

Southwestern Salad

Serve this spicy salad alone or as a filling for whole grain tortillas or your own homemade flatbread (see page 253). A dollop of homemade guacamole and organic lowfat sour cream is a nice substitute for the cilantro-lime dressing.

Makes 6 main-course servings

Leaves from 1 head romaine lettuce or red leaf lettuce, torn into
    small pieces
1 cup fresh or thawed frozen corn kernels
1 red bell pepper, seeded, deveined, and diced
1 yellow bell pepper, seeded, deveined, and diced
1 cucumber, peeled, seeded, and diced
1 large avocado, peeled, pitted, and diced
1 (15-ounce) can black beans, drained and rinsed
1 (15-ounce) can pinto beans, drained and rinsed
½ cup chopped red onion
¼ cup black olives, pitted and chopped

¼ cup shredded extra-sharp Cheddar cheese
1 teaspoon salt
½ teaspoon freshly ground black pepper
½ cup Cilantro-Lime Dressing (recipe follows)

In a salad bowl, combine all the ingredients except the dressing.
Add the dressing and toss to coat evenly.

Cilantro-Lime Dressing

Makes about ½ cup

¼ cup plain nonfat yogurt
¼ cup lowfat sour cream
2 teaspoons minced fresh cilantro
½ teaspoon grated lime zest
Juice of 1 lime
½ teaspoon sea salt
½ teaspoon freshly ground black pepper

In a small bowl, combine all the ingredients and stir to blend.
Use immediately, or cover and refrigerate for up to 3 days.

ACKNOWLEDGMENTS

IN NO PARTICULAR ORDER, I would like to thank the following people:

Janet Bray Attwood and Chris Attwood, for sharing their wonderful book, *The Passion Test*, with me.

Matthew Kelly, for sharing his enlightening books and putting me in contact with my agent.

My agent, Joe Durepos, for challenging me and working with me on my book proposal even though I didn't have the faintest idea what one was.

Jason Gardner and Kristen Cashman, my editors, for being willing to work with a first-time author, for their outstanding editorial input, and for making this book far better than the original manuscript I sent to them.

Kim Corbin, my publicist, for having so many great ideas about book promotion and for amusing me and keeping me focused.

Tracy Pitts, for her work on the cover design.

Tona Pearce Myers, for designing the interior of my book.

Marc Allen, Munro Magruder, Monique Muhlenkamp, Ami Parkerson, and all the other down-to-earth but talented and hardworking people that I've had the pleasure of meeting and working with at New World Library.

Bill Horton, for lengthy book chats over coffee and for recommending Matthew Kelly's book to me.

My sister, Kelly, for letting me share her stories, and for teaching me about the "science" part of healthy eating.

My dear friend "Stupid" (who is now eating and living healthfully), for being my favorite person to shop for denim with.

All the warm and kind people I met in Texas who treated me like family.

My Mom, Kathryn, for never telling us kids what to eat or how to live healthfully, but showing us instead.

My Dad, Steven, for going along with Mom and for passing on to me the ability to work hard but to laugh even harder.

Both my parents, for being exemplary people, for being my sun, my wind, and the most solid foundation possible, and for always putting our family first.

Aaron, Bryant, Deb, Ericka, Erin, Karen, Kari, Kathy, Katie, Meredith, Mimi, Niki, Patti, Sandy, and Teisha for either reading early drafts of my manuscript or being the first to place preorders of my book or in many cases, both.

All the people who reviewed my book, for taking the time to offer me their feedback.

Kelly's and my recipe testers, Karyn, Lisa, Mindy, and Sandy.

Bryant, for his unyielding support, friendship, and love.

And finally, to the two people who take up an enormous amount of my heart, my children, Stephanie and Cameron, who are proud of me no matter how many harebrained ideas I have because they know that every once in a while, I follow through "big-time" on one of them. Nothing else I do will ever compare to the joy of being your mom. I am grateful that you already know that. Thanks, kids. I love you.

ENDNOTES

Each note corresponds to the page number listed in the left-hand column. All websites were accessed on November 25, 2008.

INTRODUCTION

1   *"This is a really volcanic ensemble you're wearing, it's really marvelous!"*: The Internet Movie Database, "Memorable quotes for *Pretty in Pink* (1986)," www.imdb.com/title/tt0091790/quotes.

5   *With 142 million overweight or obese adult Americans*: American Heart Association, "Statistical Fact Sheet — Risk Factors, 2008 Update: Overweight and Obesity — Statistics," www.american heart.org/downloadable/heart/1197994908531FS16OVR08.pdf.

18   *"provide a ballpark idea of where you want your body to be"*: Mehmet C. Oz, MD, and Michael F. Roizen, MD, "The You Docs," *Oregonian*, June 25, 2008.

19   *according to Francisco Lopez-Jimenez, MD*: MarketWatch.com, "September 2008 Mayo Clinic Women's HealthSource Highlights Normal Weight Obesity, Regular Exercise and Cholesterol," www.marketwatch.com/news/story/september-2008-mayo -clinic-womens/story.aspx?guid=%7B92D9765C -8D7F-4925-8031-11857B77EF84%7D&dist=hppr.

21   *"Try not. Do...or do not. There is no try"*: The Internet Movie Database, "Memorable quotes for *Star Wars: Episode V — The Empire Strikes Back* (1980)," www.imdb.com/title/tt0080684/quotes.

21   *"There are no physical problems — only mental ones"*: Byron Katie, *Question Your Thinking, Change the World: Quotations from Byron Katie* (Carlsbad, CA: Hay House, 2007), 177.

ITEM #1: SODA POP, GUMMY BEARS, AND YOUR SWEET TOOTH

26   *"The intake of soft drinks containing high-fructose corn syrup (HFCS)"*: George A. Bray, "How Bad Is Fructose?" *American Journal of Clinical Nutrition* 86, no. 4 (October 2007): 895–96, www.ajcn.org/cgi/content/full/86/4/895.

26   *"I think it's a huge problem"*: Mark Francis Cohen, "What's Worse Than Sugar?" February 23, 2004, www.aarp.org/health/healthyliving/articles/sugar.html.

26   *"The theory goes like this"*: Kim Severson, "Sugar Coated," *San Francisco Chronicle*, February 18, 2004, www.sfgate.com/cgi-bin/article.cgi?f=/chronicle/archive/2004/02/18/FDGS24VKMH1.DTL.

26   *"after examining the evidence, that high fructose corn syrup"*: Kristen Gerencher, "Stirring the Pot with a Sugar Alternative," Market-Watch, www.marketwatch.com/News/Story/makers-high -fructose-corn-syrup/story.aspx?guid=%7B25CFEE9A %2DAED8%2D4FFB%2D8A60%2D2623F0916FD6%7D.

28   *The United States Department of Agriculture says that*: Mark Francis Cohen, "What's Worse Than Sugar?" AARP, February 23, 2004, www.aarp.org/health/healthyliving/articles/sugar.html.

28   *A half a pound per year*: Ibid.

30   *Pepsi helped fund the latest "research" on HFCS*: Kim Lengle, "Sweetener Controversy Grows," CBSNews.com, www .cbsnews.com/stories/2008/10/01/cbsnews_investigates/ main4491513.shtml.

31   *The World Health Organization recommends*: CBC News, "Cut Calories from Sugar: UN Report," www.cbc.ca/health/story/ 2003/03/03/diet_un030303.html.

32   *Only a small percentage can be absorbed by your body*: Marcelle Pick, OB/GYN NP, "Sugar Substitutes and the Potential

Dangers of Splenda," Women to Women, www.womentowomen
.com/nutritionandweightloss/splenda.asp.

33 *Splenda "contributes to obesity"*: Lynnley Browning, "New Salvo
in Splenda Skirmish," *New York Times*, September 22, 2008,
www.nytimes.com/2008/09/23/business/23splenda.html
?ex=1379908800&en=7bca2ca78aff31f9&ei=5124&partner=
permalink&exprod=permalink.

33 *According to an eight-year study*: Daniel J. DeNoon, "Diet Soda
Drinkers Gain Weight," CBSnews.com, June 13, 2005, www.cbs
news.com/stories/2005/06/13/health/webmd/main701408.shtm.

34 *"Our bodies are smarter than we think"*: Ibid.

36 *water bottle companies aren't required to test for pathogens*: Tappening
.com, "Why Tap Water?" www.tappening.com/Why_Tap_Water.

36 *America uses 17 million barrels of crude oil to produce plastic bottles*:
Eleftheria Parpis, "Tappening Breaks the Bottle Bonds," Ad-
week.com, May 7, 2008, www.adweek.com/aw/content_display/
news/agency/e311497897d7ff387520e2958497ae373bf.

36 *"Get off the bottle. Advocate tap"*: Adland, "Tappening: Obama,
McCain Drinking Problems — Wild Posters," September 18,
2008, http://commercial-archive.com/node/145555.

38 *"insulin is the hormone that opens your fat cells"*: Barbara Berkeley,
"The Case Against Calories," Refuse to Regain, May 27, 2008,
http://refusetoregain.typepad.com/my_weblog/2008/05/
the-case-against-calories.html

39 *The Mayo Clinic website says it may also assist in*: Katherine
Zeratsky, RD, LD, "Stevia: Is It Available in the United States?"
Mayo Clinic, November 15, 2007, www.mayoclinic.com/
health/stevia/AN01733.

ITEM #2: THE GREAT DEBATE

50 *"led many Americans to believe that carbohydrates are bad"*: Harvard
School of Public Health, "Carbohydrates: Good Carbs Guide the
Way," www.hsph.harvard.edu/nutritionsource/
what-should-you-eat/carbohydrates-full-story/index.html.

50 *"Our worries over the Atkins Diet"*: Robert H. Eckel, MD, "The

Atkins Diet: What It Is — What the Experts Say," WebMD,
www.webmd.com/diet/atkins-diet-what-it-is?page=4.

54   *"whole grain foods should contain the three key ingredients"*: Sally
Squires, "Guidelines Provide a Definition of Whole-Grain
Food," *Washington Post*, February 16, 2006, www.washington
post.com/wp-.dyn/content/article/2006/02/15/AR200602
1502580.html.

57   *According to RealAge.com, inflammation is "super bad"*:
RealAge.com, "The Calm, Quiet Vitamin — and Why You Need
It," May 23, 2008, www.realage.com/ct/tips/5907.

59   *That's what researchers at the University of California discovered*:
"Good News About Whole Grains," *Clean Eating* 1, no. 3
(Summer 2008): 19.

ITEM #3: ORGANICALLY SPEAKING

70   *"companies that handle or process organic food"*: Mary V. Gold,
"What Is Organic Production?" USDA National Agricultural Library, June 2007, www.nal.usda.gov/afsic/pubs/ofp/ofp.shtml.

70   *"treating the farm as an integrated whole"*: Union of Concerned
Scientists, "Sustainable Food Choices," www.ucsusa.org/food_and
_environment/sustainable_food.

72   *Care2 suggests that even though there is currently no sure way*:
Care2.org, "Genetically Engineered Food Labeling,"
September 11, 1999, www.care2.com/greenliving/genetically
-engineered-food-labeling.html.

72   *Look at the PLU codes of the produce you're buying*: The Editors of
E/The Environmental Magazine, *Green Living* (New York: Pen-
guin, 2005), 3.

72   *The editors of* Green Living *also suggest*: *Green Living*, 12.

73   *For coffee, the Rainforest Alliance certifies thousands of farms*:
Rainforest Alliance, "Rainforest Alliance Certified Coffee,"
www.rainforest-alliance.org/cafe/english.html.

74   *"refrigerator trucks belching carbon-dioxide"*: Joanna Pearlstein,
"Surprise! Conventional Agriculture Can Be Easier on the
Planet," *Wired* 16.06, May 19, 2008, www.wired.com/science/
planetearth/magazine/16-06/ff_heresies_03organics.

76   *"This outgassing is sufficiently toxic to kill pet birds"*: Jane Houlihan, Kris Thayer, and Jennifer Klein, "Canaries in the Kitchen: Teflon Toxicosis," Environmental Working Group, May 2003, www.ewg.org/reports/toxictcflon.

77   ShopSmart *magazine (from the folks at* Consumer Reports*)*: ConsumerReports.org, "When It Pays to Buy Organic," February 2006, www.consumerreports.org/cro/food/diet-nutrition/organic-products/organic-products-206/overview/index.htm.

ITEM #4: FAST FOOD IS FAT FOOD

81   *"If you have one sick cow in the batch"*: Eric Schlosser, "Fast Food Nation: Meat and Potatoes," *Rolling Stone* 794 (September 1998), available at www.ericsecho.org/investigation2.htm.

82   *E. coli found in hamburgers is responsible for deaths*: Ibid.

FOOD FOR THOUGHT: FAILED ATTEMPTS

90   *"The notion that there is such a thing as a proper beginning"*: Patricia Ryan Madson, *Improv Wisdom* (New York: Bell Tower, 2005), 53.

90   *"Once it is under way, any task seems smaller"*: Madson, *Improv Wisdom*, 59.

ITEM #5: MIXERS, MODERATION, AND MARGARITAS

91   *Research conducted at the University of Barcelona*: Amy Norton, "Wine May Calm Inflammation in Blood Vessels," Reuters.com, November 27, 2007, www.reuters.com/article/healthNews/idUSCOL76345520071127.

91   *The* New York Times *has more good news*: Tara Parker-Pope, "Red Wine May Curb Fat Cells," NYTimes.com, June 17, 2008, http://well.blogs.nytimes.com/2008/06/17/red-wine-may-curb-fat-cells/?scp=2&sq=red%20wine&st=cse; and Nicholas Wade, "New Signs Seen That Red Wine May Slow Aging," *New York Times*, June 4, 2008, www.nytimes.com/2008/06/04/health/research/04aging.html?_r=1&oref=slogin.

92   *"Cranberry juice contains high levels of organic acids"*: Health-Doc.com, "Cranberry Juice to the Rescue," www.health-doc.com/healtharticles/cranberry-juice.html.

93   *"If you are thin, physically active, don't smoke"*: Harvard School of Public Health, "Alcohol: Balancing Risks and Benefits," www.hsph.harvard.edu/nutritionsource/what-should-you-eat/alcohol-full-story/index.html.

ITEM #6: FOO-FOO COFFEE DRINKS

98   *A study at Purdue University says adding a squeeze of lemon juice*: "Lemon-Aid," *Clean Eating* 1, no. 3 (Summer 2008): 18.

99   *"loss of sleep alters the complex metabolic pathways"*: ScienceDaily.com, "Sleeping Less May Be Related to Weight Gain," January 11, 2005, www.sciencedaily.com/releases/2005/01/050111092501.htm.

99   *Research in the journal* Cell Metabolism *found that*: "Sleep, Wake, Eat," *Clean Eating* 1, no. 3 (Summer 2008): 16.

101   *The Mayo Clinic website cautions that*: Mayo Clinic, "Caffeine: How Much Is Too Much?" March 8, 2007, www.mayoclinic.com/health/caffeine/NU00600.

101   *"Studies consistently show that coffee and caffeine"*: Mehmet C. Oz, MD, and Michael F. Roizen, MD, "Crazy for Coffee: Am I Drinking Too Much Coffee?" *Reader's Digest*, July 2006, www.rd.com/living-healthy/health-iq-health-benefits-of-coffee/article27530.html.

101   *I read in* Parade *magazine recently*: Joy Bauer, "Eight Food Myths Busted," *Parade*, August 31, 2008, p. 12.

ITEM #7: THE MOST IMPORTANT MEAL OF THE DAY

103   *"Break the fast to shed the pounds"*: WebMD.com, "The Most Important Meal of the Day," www.webmd.com/diet/guide/most-important-meal.

106   *Even the beloved and trusted pediatrician Dr. Spock*: CNN.com, "Dr. Spock's Call for Vegetarian Diet Sparks Meaty Debate," www.cnn.com/HEALTH/9806/20/dr.spock; and Jane Brody, "Final Advice from Dr. Spock: Eat Only All Your Vegetables,"

New York Times, June 11, 1998, http://query.nytimes.com/gst/fullpage.html?res=9C07E4DD173CF933A15755C0A96E9582 60&partner=rssnyt&emc=rss.

106 *The Harvard School of Public Health presents a balanced view*: Harvard School of Public Health, "Calcium and Milk: What's Best for Your Bones?" www.hsph.harvard.edu/nutritionsource/what -should-you-eat/calcium-full-story/index.html.

107 *Dr. Oz says vitamin D also helps reduce the risk of immune disorders*: Mehmet Oz, MD, and Michael Roizen, MD, "Unhealthy Practices That Won't Kill You," Esquire.com, April 30, 2008, www .esquire.com/features/better-man/dont-worry-0508.

107 *Michael Holick, MD, author of* The UV Advantage: Mike Adams, "Vitamin D Myths, Facts, and Statistics," NaturalNews.com, www.naturalnews.com/003069.html.

108 *According to a study published in* Molecular Systems Biology: ScienceDaily.com, "Probiotics Affect Metabolism, Says New Study," January 16, 2008, www.sciencedaily.com/releases/ 2008/01/080115085347.htm.

109 *Pomegranate juice is supposedly good for men's prostate health*: Erik Castle, MD, "Pomegranate Juice: A Cure for Cancer?" www.mayoclinic.com/health/pomegranate-juice/AN01477.

109 *Lemonade has been shown to slow the development*: Daniel J. De-Noon, "Lemonade Helps Kidney Stones," WebMD.com, May 24, 2006, www.webmd.com/kidney-stones/news/20060524/ lemonade-helps-kidney-stones.

109 *A high concentration of cranberry juice*: ScienceDaily.com, "Cranberries Help Combat Urinary Tract Infections in Women, Researcher Finds," January 14, 2008, www.sciencedaily.com/ releases/2008/01/080110123918.htm.

FOOD FOR THOUGHT: GOING TO EXTREMES

111 *Research at the Indiana University School of Medicine*: Sound Medicine, "Yo-Yo Dieting," August 28, 2005, www.soundmedicine .iu.edu/segment.php4?seg=586.

111   *The* American Journal of Clinical Nutrition *found the same*: Ibid.

113   *"If a person with anorexia becomes severely malnourished"*: Mayo Clinic, "Anorexia Nervosa," December 20, 2007, www.mayo clinic.com/health/anorexia/DS00606.

ITEM #8: MEAT ME IN THE MIDDLE

118   *"If 10,000 people gave up steak once every seven days"*: Jen Boulden, "My Green Life: The Nice Know-It-All" *Domino* 4, no. 1 (February 2008), http://www.dominomag.com/magazine/2007/12/jen_boulden?currentPage=2.

119   *"about two to five times more grain is required"*: Mark Bittman, "Re-thinking the Meat-Guzzler," *New York Times,* January 27, 2008, www.nytimes.com/2008/01/27/weekinreview/27bittman.html?pagewanted=1&_r=2.

119   *"Then imagine the room filled"*: Frances Moore Lappé, *Diet for a Small Planet* (New York: Ballantine, 1980), 14.

121   *A Harvard School of Public Health study shows*: Harvard School of Public Health, "New Study Shows the Benefits of Eating Fish Greatly Outweigh the Risks," October 17, 2006, www.hsph.harvard.edu/news/press-releases/2006-releases/press10172006.html.

122   *"wild fish caught from healthy, well-managed populations"*: Environmental Defense Fund, "Eco-Best Fish," www.edf.org/page.cfm?tagID=15890.

123   *As of this writing, the current list of "Eco-Best" is as follows*: Environmental Defense Fund, "Make Smart Choices When Eating Seafood," www.edf.org/page.cfm?tagID=1521.

124   *"chickens on today's factory farms"*: GoVeg.com, "The Chicken Flesh Industry," www.goveg.com/factoryFarming_chickens_flesh.asp.

ITEM #9: YOUR MOM WAS SO RIGHT

127   *Bauer reminds us to read labels carefully*: Joy Bauer, "Eight Food Myths Busted," *Parade,* August 31, 2008, p. 12.

128   *The Harvard School of Public Health website says*: Harvard School

of Public Health, "Antioxidants: Beyond the Hype," www
.hsph.harvard.edu/nutritionsource/what-should-you-eat/
antioxidants/#evidence.

ITEM #10: GOT FAT?

133 *"something that interferes with the metabolic processes of life"*: Eric
Armstrong, "What's Wrong with Partially Hydrogenated Oils?"
www.treelight.com/health/nutrition/PartiallyHydrogenated
Oils.html.

135 *coconut flakes, milk, and oil contain lauric acid*: Nina Planck, "What
America Eats: Six Superfoods to Know," *Parade*, March 30, 2008,
www.ninaplanck.com/index.php?article=superfoods.

135 *"some foods that are rich in saturated fat"*: Katherine Tallmadge,
"So Saturated," *Washington Post*, June 2, 2004, www.washington
post.com/wp-dyn/articles/A5980-2004Jun1.html.

135 *"all saturated fat speeds up aging"*: Mehmet C. Oz, MD, and
Michael F. Roizen, MD, "Don't Fall for This Celeb Health
Trend," RealAge.com, http://realage.typepad.com/youdocs
daily/2008/11/dont-fall-for-this-celeb-health-trend.html.

136 *The American Heart Association recommends*: American Heart
Association, "Saturated Fats," www.americanheart.org/presenter
.jhtml?identifier=3045790.

136 *"The key to a healthy diet is to substitute good fats for bad fats"*:
Harvard School of Public Health, "Choose Healthy Fats, Limit
Saturated Fat, and Avoid Trans Fat," www.hsph.harvard.edu/
nutritionsource/what-should-you-eat/fats-and-cholesterol.

136 *the number one killer of both women and men*: DHHS Centers for
Disease Control and Prevention, "Heart Disease Is the Number
One Cause of Death," www.cdc.gov/DHDSP/announcements/
american_heart_month.htm.

137 *"When plaque breaks apart, it can cause a heart attack or stroke"*:
Harvard School of Public Health, "Fats and Cholesterol: Out
with the Bad, In with the Good," www.hsph.harvard.edu/
nutritionsource/what-should-you-eat/fats-full-story/index.html.

137 *The* American Journal of Clinical Nutrition *reported*: "Benefits of

Berries," *Body + Soul*, August 2007, www.wholeliving.com/article/
benefits-of-berries?autonomy_kw=hdl%20levels%20berries.

ITEM #11: LEAN AND GREEN

143 *Even better, five hundred tons of used items*: Freecycle.org, "History and
Background Information," www.freecycle.org/about/background.

144 *The* Wall Street Journal *reported that the United States consumes*:
Ellen Gamerman, "An Inconvenient Bag," *Wall Street Journal*,
September 26, 2008, http://online.wsj.com/article/
SB122238422541876879.html.

ITEM #12: TEN A.M. AND THREE P.M.

151 *The Mayo Clinic says that 77 percent of our sodium intake*: Mayo
Clinic, "Sodium: Are You Getting Too Much?" May 23, 2008,
www.mayoclinic.com/health/sodium/NU00284.

ITEM #13: I LIKE THE WAY YOU MOVE

159 *By substituting twenty minutes a day of walking for driving*: Iowa State
University Department of Food Science and Human Nutrition,
"Walking Facts and Benefits," www.fshn.hs.iastate.edu/nutrition
clinic/handouts/WalkingFactsBenefits.pdf.

ITEM #16: EATING AWAY FROM HOME

204 *one Ikea meatball has forty calories and three grams of fat*: The Daily
Plate, www.thedailyplate.com/nutrition/search/?q=ikea+meat
ball&x=59&y=10.

204 *The nachos at Target contain 1,101 calories*: CalorieKing.com,
http://www.calorieking.com/foods/calories-in-restaurant
-international-foods-nachos-w-cheese_f-Y2lkPTM5JmJpZDoxO
TkzJmZpZDoxMTI4MzQmZWlkPTMoNzE4NDYxNCZwb3M
9MSZwYXI9JmtleT1oYXJnZXQgbmFjaG9z.html.

INDEX

INDEX

composting, 84
convenience stores, 204–5
cooking sprays, 75, 138
co-ops, food, 78
cortisol, 101
coupons, 77
cranberry juice, 92
cravings, 37, 87
creamers, coffee, 97–98
Cream of Pumpkin Soup, 256–57
Crunchy Cobb Salad, 262–63
Cucumber Sandwiches, 250

D

dairy products, 105–9, 216–17
dark chocolate, 135–36, 153
decision making, 16
deli food, 202
dementia, 135
depression, 107
dessert, 39–40, 180
diabetes, 51, 53, 107
    type 2, 19, 39, 114
Diet for a Small Planet (Lappé), 119
dieting, 111–13
digestion, 54
dining companions, 161–65
doughnuts, 188
drinks, 218
    alcoholic, 91–95
    Bellini, 233
    caffeinated, 97–102
    Mojito, 231

E

eating
    away from home, 177–206

companions, 161–65
    purposeful, 20
Eatwellguide.org, 75
Eckel, Robert H., 50
E. coli, 82
edamame, 189–90
eggs, 104–5, 217
    Egg Salad, 253–54
    Garden Walnut Scramble,
        231–32
    Mediterranean Scramble, 228–29
    South-of-the-Border Scramble,
        229–30
    whites, 105
endosperm, 54
Energy Bars, 236–38
Equal, 37
erythritol, 32
essential fatty acids, 134
exercise, 19–20, 157–61

F

fairs, 182
fair-trade movement, 70–71
falafel, 199
farmers' markets, 74
Farmers' Market Salad, 263–64
fast food, 29–30, 81–85
fat
    essential fatty acids, 134, 138
    good vs. bad, 133–39
    insulin and, 38, 52
    in meat, 120
    omega-3 fatty acids, 120, 121,
        138–39, 189–90, 201
    saturated, 135, 136
    trans fatty acids, 133–35

INDEX

INDEX

ABOUT THE AUTHOR

KAMI GRAY IS A TV WARDROBE STYLIST and art director who discovered a simple system for staying slender and healthy while she was a young college student. She has designed costumes and sets for over a hundred commercials, including national spots for Toyota, Nike, Discover Card, Blockbuster, and AOL. Kami has worked for TV shows, including *House*, *Veronica Mars*, and *Hell's Kitchen*, and with Hollywood actors, including Kristen Bell, Jenny McCarthy, Hugh Laurie, Taye Diggs, Patty Duke, Shannen Doherty, and Sean Astin. She's the single mom of a college freshman and a high school senior and lives in Portland, Oregon. Kami is available to inspire, motivate, and educate groups, companies, and organizations about healthy eating. Her websites are www.kamigray.com, www.thedenimdiet.com, and http://blog.kamigray.com/